THE KETO LIFE FOR BEGINNERS

KICKSTART YOUR KETO WEIGHT LOSS JOURNEY IN 10 DAYS

JANE ARDANA

Table of Contents

Chapter 1: How It Works

There are so many different diet plans out there, it can be confusing and overwhelming when you are deciding which one would work best for you. Some of these diets are trends or fads and not something that can be maintained long-term, others might make you feel hungry all the time, which as you know, does not make for a happy life. This is one of the reasons the ketogenic diet stands apart from the rest, it will help you lose weight, while also letting you feel satisfied. You are not starving your body of calories or fat on the ketogenic diet.

What Does Ketogenic Mean?

When you eat a more traditional diet that is higher in carbohydrates your body produces glucose and insulin. Glucose is the body's first choice of energy source because it is the easiest for the body to convert. Insulin's role is to process the glucose that is in your bloodstream by taking it around the body. When this happens, it means that the fats in your body are not needed, since they are not the energy source. The fat still has to go somewhere though, so the body stores it for later use.

When you lower your carbohydrate intake, your body will enter into a state known as ketosis, which is where the word ketogenic comes from. Ketosis is what the body initiates when food consumption is low, it is a natural process that is meant to help the body survive. During ketosis the liver will break down fats and produce ketones which can also be used as fuel for the body, but only if glucose is in short supply. Remember, glucose is the body's first choice, so it will only use something else when glucose is not an option. It is not because it can't or that is not healthy, when using ketones as fuel, the body just has to work a little harder.

The goal of the ketogenic diet is to get your body to switch from using glucose as its fuel supply, to ketones, which you would get from the breakdown of fat. Therefore, your body would be getting all its energy from fat. As your insulin levels lower, your body's fat burning abilities will increase. For most people, this happens very quickly and quite dramatically. One of the benefits of this diet is how easy it becomes to burn through stored fat, which obviously helps if weight loss is your main goal.

The quickest way to enter ketosis is by fasting, however that cannot be maintained without harmful effects. The ketogenic diet can be followed indefinitely, while still allowing the body to enter ketosis. This is not a diet that deals with calorie counting, meaning you cannot eat what ever you want as long as you don't go over your caloric limit. Keeping your carbohydrate intake low, it is suggested no more than 20 or 30g of net carbohydrates is how you will be successful. However, the less you consume, the more dramatic your weight loss will be.

What is a Net Carb?

Net carb = Total dietary carbohydrate − Total fiber

Let's assume you want to eat one cup of broccoli, which contains 6g of total carbohydrates and 2g of fiber. To find the net carbs, you would then take the 6g minus the 2g, leaving you with 4g, which is the net carb amount.

Your ketogenic diet should be made of around 70 percent fats, 25 percent proteins, and only 5 percent should be carbohydrates. This is why it is so important to pay attention to what you are putting into your body and whether or not it will prevent you from entering ketosis.

The ketogenic diet will yield impressive results, but only if you stick to it. When you eat too many carbohydrates, your body will have the insulin it needs to use as fuel, meaning the fat will be stored instead of burned. The secret to a successful ketogenic diet is to plan-out what you will eat, this will not only reduce your stress, but it will also keep you on the right track.

Just like any diet or lifestyle change, it will take time for you to properly adjust to it, but you can do it. One of the best things you can do for yourself is to keep an open mind and allow yourself the time necessary to acclimate. Rushing things before you are fully prepared will not help you, it will only cause you added stress which will probably lead to failure. To prevent this from happening, it is crucial that you find what works for you while still adhering to the diet.

Some people prefer to prep their meals a head of time, especially breakfast and lunch since they often take it with them to work. Other people like to write out their meals like a menu and stick with their ideas. You don't have to do this, but it definitely make things easier on you, especially in the beginning.

When you are on a special diet like this one, it probably won't take you very long to see how much easier it is to cook at home. Being in complete control of your food is crucial to remaining in ketosis and losing weight. That being said, if you do decide to go to a restaurant, make sure to ask any appropriate questions involving your order. Being specific about what foods are cooked in or how they are prepared will help make sure you are sticking to your diet.

Just remember, you are not going to be hungry, your body is learning to depend a different fuel for energy. That takes some time to get accustomed to, so be patient with yourself and find what works best for you. For instance, if you prefer to prep all of your meals for the week on Sunday, do it. However, if you work the night shift and enjoy cooking when you arrive home in the morning, feel free to do it that way, just find what works for you and stick to it.

Chapter 2: All about Food

Starting a new diet can be frustrating and irritating, especially if you think you are sticking to the rules, but are not seeing any positive results. This is why it is so important to know exactly what you are allowed to eat what you are not. If you don't know what foods are acceptable and are not knowledgeable about your diet, you won't be successful, regardless of the effort you are putting forth. So, make it easy on yourself and learn which foods you should eat and which you should avoid.

The best way to think of the ketogenic diet is to think real, whole foods. Anything that is prepackaged or processed is full of net carbohydrates and is off limits. This means staying away from pastas, cereals, breads, and cakes. Fruits and vegetables also contain carbohydrates so it is important that you also keep track of these net carbs as well. You already know that your diet is going to consist of mostly healthy fats, but you might understand what that means exactly. Well, first, not all fats are equal, some are definitely better for you than others and it is crucial that you know the difference.

Fats, Good and Bad

Foods contain different types of fats, but are categorized by what they contain the most of. For instance, butter is considered a saturated fat because it contains 60 percent saturated fat. As you move forward with your diet you will quickly understand the role fats play, without them you would be hungry all the time and would be left feeling unsatisfied.

Saturated Fats – These are known as essential to our health as they help to keep our immune systems healthy. In addition to helping with the immune system, this fat will also help balance hormone levels and maintain a normal bone density. This type of fat has a bad reputation and time and again has been included in the 'bad for you' category, but many different studies have shown that they are important and necessary for a healthy body. Meats, butter, and eggs all have saturated fats in them.

Polyunsaturated Fats – This is the type of fat that is commonly found in vegetable oils, and for a long time they were thought to be beneficial. However, that is not the case as they are often over processed, for instance, "heart healthy" margarines have been linked to heart disease. Yet, polyunsaturated fats that are natural such as those found in fish actually help to lower cholesterol, so it is important to know the difference and not get them confused. This is why real, natural foods are so important because the fats they contain are much better for you than their highly processed counterparts.

Monounsaturated Fats – This is an accepted healthy fat, as it improves insulin resistance and cholesterol levels. This type of fat is found in both sunflower and olive oils, both of which are common and easy to incorporate into your diet.

Trans Fats – You probably already know that trans fats are not good for you, they do not occur in natural fatty foods, only processed fatty foods. That is an important distinction, because this type of fat is created from chemicals that are used to extend a food's shelf-life. For instance, the hydrogenation process is when hydrogen is added to these fats which changes their chemical make-up. Even if a label does not say it contains trans fats, if it says hydrogenated on it, avoid it.

When you are doing your grocery shopping, try to purchase organic products and grass-fed proteins. Avoid canned or frozen fruits and vegetables too, but it is understandable that some people just do not have the financial means to do this, so be cautious and make sure you read all the labels. The next chapters are going to contain some recipes that you can try, but as you progress with your diet, you will see how easy it is to incorporate healthy fats into your meals. This will help you feel satisfied and will help you stay fuller longer.

Fats:

Avocado
Beef Tallow

Chicken Fat
Macadamia Nuts
Ghee
Butter
Non-hydrogenated Lard
Mayonnaise – read the label and make sure it does not have added carbs.
Red palm oil
Peanut butter
Olive oil
Coconut oil

Proteins:

Fish – Try to purchase wild caught if available, this can include salmon, trout, catfish, halibut, cod, flounder, mackerel, tuna, and snapper.

Shellfish – Crab, oysters, mussels, squid, lobster, scallops, and clams.

Whole Eggs – Opt for free-range if you can, local organic farmers often have them cheaper than your local grocery stores. When it comes to preparation you have many different options such as boiled, poached, scrambled, deviled, and fried.

Meat – Grass-fed typically has a higher fatty acid count, so opt for grass-fed when given the opportunity. Goat, lamb, veal, beef, and other wild game are all good choices.

Pork – You can eat nearly any type of pork, just make sure to read the label to make sure there are no added sugars.

Poultry – Pheasant, quail, chicken, and duck are all acceptable, but choose free range and organic if it is possible.

Sausage and Bacon – This can still be an acceptable and even beneficial protein as long as you choose it wisely, make sure there are no extra fillers and that it is not cured in sugar.

Peanut Butter – Choose natural peanut butter, but make sure to read the label carefully, even the most natural peanut butter can contain high amounts of carbohydrates, a better alternative is macadamia nut butter.

Vegetables

The best vegetables to eat on the ketogenic diet are those that are leafy and grow above ground. Again, if you can eat organic, try to do so as there will less pesticides used in the growing process, but if you can't try not to worry too much. Studies have shown that both non-organic and organic vegetables have the same nutritional qualities.

Of course vegetables are good for you, but some are better than others in terms of the ketogenic diet. For instance, some vegetables are high in sugar and lower in important nutrients, these are the types of vegetables that you want to either cut out altogether or consume only in very small portions. The best vegetables for this diet are those that are low in carbohydrates and high in nutrients, such as kale and anything green leafy that resembles it. These types of veggies are also easy to include in meals and they really pack a powerful nutrition punch as well.

Remember, vegetables also contain carbohydrates, so make sure you are keeping track throughout the day so you stay well within the acceptable limit. The following is a list of vegetables and their net carbohydrates by ounce.

Avocado - .6

Broccoli – 1.1

Baby Carrots – 1.5

Cauliflower - .5

Celery - .3

Cucumber – 1

Green Beans – 1.3

Mushrooms - .6

Green Onion – 1.3

White Onion – 2.1

Green Pepper - .8

Romaine Lettuce - .3

Butterhead Lettuce - .3

Shallots – 3.9

Snow Peas – 2.8

Spinach - .4

Acorn Squash – 2.9

Butternut Squash – 2.1

Spaghetti Squash – 1.4

Tomato - .8

As you begin making your own meal plans, simply add up the net carbohydrates between the different foods so you have an idea of how many you are consuming from that meal. This will get easier over time, you can even try writing it down in the beginning until you get more comfortable keeping track.

Dairy

Dairy products are also acceptable as long as there is no added sugars or other additives. It is best to go choose full fat, raw, and organic.

Sour Cream

Cottage Cheese

Heavy Whipping Cream

Hard and Soft Cheeses (Cream cheese, cheddar, mozzarella, mascarpone, etc)

You probably are guessed what is going to be said next, but it really can't be stressed enough, make sure you read the labels. Many cheeses are low in net carbohydrates as it is, but if you are in doubt either read the label or as the person behind the counter.

Nuts and Seeds

Seeds and nuts are a great way to add healthy fats to your diet and make a wonderful and convenient snack. It is best to eat them when they are roasted, this process removes any anti-nutrients. It is also important to note that there is a difference between a nut and a legume, nuts are allowed, while legumes are generally not permitted. Oddly enough, based on the name, a peanut is a legume and should be avoided. Here is a list of acceptable nuts and seeds:

Macadamias, walnuts, and almonds, all of these should be eaten in moderation, but their carbohydrate count is relatively low.

Pistachios and cashews are both higher in carbohydrates, but do contain healthy fats, so make sure you keep careful track of them.

Tip: Seed and nut flower are good alternatives to white or wheat flour, but try not to make this a staple in your diet because nuts are high in Omega-6 fatty acids, so be careful with over eating them because it can lead to weight gain and slow your progress.

Beverages

When you start your ketogenic diet, you will notice that it will have a natural diuretic effect, which means hydration is even more important. Also, if you are someone who is prone to bladder pain or urinary tract infections, you will need to be even more diligent when it comes to hydrating. It is suggested that you not only drink the recommended eight glasses of water each day, more in addition. Our bodies are made up of 2/3 water, so make sure you are keeping it happy and hydrated. Drink appropriate liquids like it is going out of style!

Water, drink it. Drink a lot of it.

Coffee, with heavy cream and no sugar, it is fine in moderation.

Tea, also no added sugar and if you like it with milk make sure it is raw and whole fat or use heavy cream.

Sweeteners

Of course it is best to avoid anything that is sweet, but for some of us with a sweet tooth, this would just make us miserable. That being said, if you have a sweet craving that you can't seem to deny, choose an artificial sweetener and try not to do this often. Liquid sweeteners are better since there are no added binders like in the powder forms that have carbohydrates.

Stevia

Sucralose

Monk Fruit

Erythirol

Xylitol

Spices

When it comes to what you eat, you want it to be flavorful and satisfying, most of which will come from the addition of spices. However, many spices contain carbohydrates, so it is important that you keep track of the amounts of you are using and add those amounts to your carbohydrate total for your meal. You can use nearly any dry spices you prefer, just make sure you look up the carbohydrate content, no one wants your food to be boring and bland. Some spices have more carbs than others, such as cinnamon, garlic powder, allspice, bay leaves, ginger, and cardamom, so if those are staples in your cooking, make sure you are keeping accurate track.

Watch Out For

Fruit – Limit your fruit content because fruit is high in natural sugars and therefore carbohydrates. Many people use berries in desserts or as snacks, but only in small portions and not very often. If you choose to do this, be cautious of raspberries, cranberries, and blueberries.

Tomato – Food companies are very good at making their products look healthier than they really are. Tomatoes do have natural sugars in them, but when you buy tomato based products additional sugar is often added. That doesn't mean you can't use canned tomato sauces or diced tomatoes, just make sure you read the labels.

Peppers – Most of us do not think of peppers as being full of sugars, green has the last amount of sugars compared to red or yellow.

Diet Sodas – You can still drink diet soda, just pay close attention to how much you are drinking and try to limit yourself if you are soda dependent. Some people have reported that they were knocked out of ketosis from consuming too much artificial sweetener, so just keep that in mind when you are considering a diet soda.

Salt – Since the ketogenic diet acts as a natural diuretic, you will see that your body does not retain salt the same way it did before. This means that salt and other electrolytes are flushed from the body very quickly, this can lead to many different health issues such as panic attacks and heart palpitations. To prevent this from happening you can include salted bone broth into your diet or you can use what is known as a light salt that is a combination of both salt and potassium. Most people also choose to take a supplement for anything they think are not getting enough of from their diet.

Water – When you think you have consumed enough water, drink a little more. Your body is going through some huge changes and part of that is flushing out liquids faster than before, so to keep yourself healthy it is a good idea to drink water, a lot of water.

In The Beginning

If this your first time embarking on a low carbohydrate diet, there are some things you need to know. Your body is doing to go through what is known as detox symptoms, this is perfectly natural, but uncomfortable. Remember, you are retraining your body, that doesn't happen without consequences. However, don't be discouraged, they only last for a few days and no matter how bad it feels, you can and will get through it.

These withdrawal symptoms are commonly referred to as the "keto flu," which sounds much worse than it is. Just keep telling yourself that the first three days are the hardest and it will get much easier after. Here is a list of the symptoms:

Irritability

Fatigue

Dizziness

Intense Cravings

Basically, your body is acting like an unruly child who wants sugar, because it has become so accustomed to it. For those who are transitioning from a very carbohydrate dense diet the symptoms will be much worse than others, it just depends on the person's body. Just don't give up. There are some things you can do to help cope with the negative side effects by increasing your water intake. When the very intense cravings hit, and they will, give your body something to eat, just not what it wants, try bacon or cheese. You are not denying yourself food, just distracting it from craving carbohydrates, until you adjust, distraction is the key to success.

Benefits

Now that you just read about the negative side effects, you might be feeling even more overwhelmed than before. However, the benefits of the ketogenic diet far outweighs the negative. Here is a list of the benefits:

Less appetite – After your body has had time to adjust to ketosis, your appetite will just naturally be reduced. This will also eventually lead to less calorie intake too.

Weight Loss – Not only will you lose weight on this diet, but not all fat is the same. When you hold more fat in the abdominal area, this can cause many different health issues, even increasing your risk of heart disease. The ketogenic diet will help you lose weight in the abdominal area, and usually rather quickly, this will help those who are risk for type 2 diabetes as well as heart disease.

Blood Pressure – The ketogenic diet helps to reduce high blood pressure and is often suggested by doctors for this reason.

The Brain – Some parts of the brain can only use glucose which is why our liver will create glucose from protein when we do not eat carbohydrates. However, most of the brain is capable of using ketones as fuel. Allowing the brain to use ketones as fuel has helped many children and adults alike with epilepsy. Currently, scientists are looking into a connection between the ketogenic diet and Alzheimer's disease.

Now, you have an idea of what you are going to be eating and how to count the net carbohydrates in the foods. When you first start out, keep very close track of your portion sizes so you can keep an accurate record of the net carbs. If you are choosing to remain under 20 net carbohydrates a day, then make sure to include not only the ingredients from the meal you are eating, but also from the beverage and even the spices. You will want to do this for each meal so you know for sure you are not exceeding your limit.

This is probably not going to come very easily in the beginning, but rest assured, it will get easier for you. Also, after you stick to the diet for a couple of weeks, you will already start to see results and nothing works to motivate quite like seeing the desired results. Even if it feels like you just can't keep going, or you want to give up, don't, it was hard for nearly everyone in the beginning. You are going through something huge, retraining your brain and learning to control your cravings. Chances are, you are also breaking some bad habits as well, so give yourself the necessary time to fully adjust.

Chapter 3: Ketogenic Breakfasts

This is a collection of ketogenic recipes that you can mix and match to give you a three week jump start on your diet. This will help you by taking the guess work out of what to make and it will also give you a general idea of how to prepare the correct foods for yourself. Once you start your new diet, you might find that you choose to meal prep for the week, and if that is the case, make sure your choices are able to be stored appropriately.

Many people think breakfast is one of the hardest meals to create because you can only eat so many eggs and bacon before you are craving variety. For that purpose, traditional eggs and bacon or sausage are going to be avoided, in favor of other easy and more creative options.

Egg Porridge

1/3 cup heavy cream
2 eggs
Cinnamon to taste
2 tablespoons butter
Berries, optional
Sweetener, optional

This is a ketogenic version of oatmeal or porridge, it is based on how eggs curdle and uses that grainy feel as added texture. You can choose whether or not to add berries or sweetener, depending on how many carbohydrates you are allotting yourself.

1. Combine the cream, eggs, and sweetener if you choose to use it in a small bowl and whisk the mixture together until uniform in color.
2. In a saucepan melt the butter over medium-high heat, but keep an eye on it and do not allow it to turn brown. Once the butter is melted, turn the heat to low.

3. Add the cream and egg mixture to the butter in the saucepan, make sure you continue mixing, especially along the bottom because that is where it will start to curdle and thicken first. Once you start to see the little grains or curdles remove it from the heat.
4. Add a serving to a bowl and sprinkle the top with cinnamon and the berries if you choose.

Cream Cheese Pancakes

2 eggs
½ teaspoon cinnamon
2 ounces of cream cheese (read the label and make sure there are no added sugars)
1 teaspoon sweetener, optional
Butter, to grease pan
You will also need a blender or a food processor for this recipe.

1. Place all the ingredients into the blender or food processor and mix until smooth. Sit it aside and allow it to rest for two or three minutes, or until the bubbles are settled.
2. Grease the pan and set it on medium high heat, with the butter and pour the batter onto the pan, just like you would with traditional pancakes. Cook for two minutes and then flip, cook for an additional minute or until golden brown. Repeat this until all of the batter has been used.
3. You can eat these with sugar-free syrup, berries, or nothing at all depending on what your carbohydrate limit is.

This is a great recipe to make for large groups since it is so easy and quick. They will make a great addition to your diet and will leave you feeling full and satisfied.

Lemon Poppy Seed Muffins

2 tablespoons poppy seeds
Zest of 2 lemons

3 tablespoons lemon juice
3 large eggs
¾ cup almond flour
¼ cup flaxseed meal
1 teaspoon vanilla extract
¼ cup heavy cream
1/3 cup erythritol
1 teaspoon baking powder
¼ salted butter, melted
25 drops of liquid sweetener
Muffin pan and liners

1. Set your oven to 250F, and in a bowl combine the flaxseed meal, poppy seeds, almond flour, and erythritol.
2. Slowly pour in the eggs and heavy cream, stir constantly until the mixture is smooth and there are no lumps in the batter.
3. Once the mixture is smooth add the sweetener, vanilla extract, lemon juice, lemon zest, and baking powder. Make sure to stir this well to ensure everything is mixed together properly.
4. Put your liners in the muffin pan, or silicone molds, this batter will make 12 muffins, but if you need to you can adjust the size a little, just try not to make them too big.
5. Place your batter in the oven and bake for 18 to 20 minutes, if you want a crispier crust on the bottom, leave them in for a bit longer.
6. When they are finished baking, take them out of the oven and let them rest on the counter for around 10 minutes.

These are the perfect breakfast for people who want something they can easily take with them. If you know you are in for a busy week, these make for a great breakfast to make before your work week starts.

'McGriddle' Casserole

10 eggs
1 cup almond flour

¼ cup flaxseed meal
1 pound breakfast sausage
½ teaspoon onion powder
½ teaspoon garlic powder
¼ teaspoon sage
4 tablespoons sage
4 ounce cheddar cheese
6 tablespoons sugar free syrup
Salt and pepper to taste
Casserole pan
Parchment paper

1. Preheat the oven to 350F and put a pan on medium heat, this is for the breakfast sausage. You are going to break it up as you brown it.
2. In a large mixing bowl combine all of the dry ingredients, mix them together and then add the wet ingredients, but only put in 4 tablespoons of the syrup. Mix everything together until is uniform and smooth.
3. After your mixture is mixed well, add the cheese and stir some more.
4. Throughout this process, you should also be checking on your sausage to make sure it is not getting too brown, you just want it to be a little crispy. When it is cooked to your liking, pour it, with the fat, into the mixture and stir everything together.
5. Place the parchment paper into your casserole pan and pour the mixture into the dish. Drizzle the remaining syrup over the top of the mixture.
6. Bake for about 45 to 55 minutes, if your pan is larger and your casserole thinner, you will need to adjust the cooking time to a bit less. You want the inside to be cooked through completely though, you'll know it is when it is golden brown and looks firm.
7. When it is done cooking, remove it from the oven and gently pull out the parchment paper, slice the casserole into pieces and serve with either sugar-free ketchup, or even a little more syrup.

This is a great recipe that you can eat all week. Feel free to alter the recipe to suit your needs, for instance, if you think it is too much syrup, you can adjust the amount.

Breakfast Tacos

6 eggs
3 strips of bacon
½ avocado
1 cup shredded mozzarella, make sure it is whole milk
1 ounce shredded cheddar cheese
2 tablespoons butter
Salt and pepper to taste

1. First, you are going to cook the bacon, the easiest way is to preheat your oven to 375F and bake it for 15 to 20 minutes, but if you choose to cook it in a pan, that's fine too.
2. While the bacon is cooking, put 1/3 of a cup of mozzarella in a clean pan on medium heat. You want it to be uniform in thickness and in a circle, this is what will be your taco shell. Be patient, this takes some practice to get right, but you'll get the hang of it.
3. After about two or three minutes the edges will be brown, this is when you are going to carefully slide a spatula underneath it. If you used whole milk mozzarella this should be easy since the oils in it prevent it from sticking naturally.
4. Rest a wooden spoon over a large bowl, using either tongs or your spatula, gently drape the mozzarella over the spoon so as it hardens it will be in the shape of a crunchy taco shell. Do this to the rest of the mozzarella, which will leave you with three completed shells when finished.
5. Your next step is to cook your eggs in the butter, you can do a soft or a hard scramble, it's your preference.
6. When your eggs are finished, spoon them into each of your taco shells and add the sliced avocado on top. Then top with our

bacon, you can simply place the entire slice on each, or dice it up.

7. The final step is to sprinkle the cheddar cheese on each taco and enjoy.

This is a breakfast that helps people transition when they are craving that crunch that carbohydrates provides. So, if you find yourself craving chips or breads, this might help satisfy you. Keep in mind though, that even though these do not take too long to make, they are not like the casserole where you can make extra for the week. You are pretty much just making a serving at a time.

Brownie Muffins

¼ cup cocoa powder
1 cup flaxseed meal
½ tablespoon baking powder
1 egg
1 tablespoon cinnamon
2 tablespoons coconut oil
½ teaspoon salt
½ pumpkin puree, if canned read the label carefully
¼ sugar-free caramel syrup
1 teaspoon apple cider vinegar
¼ slivered almonds
1 teaspoon vanilla extract

1. Preheat your oven to 350F and put all the dry ingredients into a large mixing bowl.
2. In a separate mixing bowl combine all the wet ingredients and stir until uniform and smooth.
3. Gently pour the wet ingredients into the dry bowl and mix together until everything is smooth and it is smooth.
4. Put your muffin liners into your pan and spoon about ¼ cup of batter into each one, and sprinkle the almonds over the top, press them down slightly so they don't fall off. This recipe will

make 6 muffins, if you need 12, simply double all of the ingredients.

5. Place them in the oven and check on them after about 15 minutes, you will know they're done when they rise. You can eat them either cold or warm, they make the perfect addition to your morning coffee.

This is the perfect breakfast for anyone who has a sweet tooth. So, for those who are starting a low carbohydrate diet for the first time, these can help with those intense sweet carb cravings. You should not feel hungry and unsatisfied on your diet and this is a great way to make sure that doesn't happen.

These breakfasts can be mixed and matched throughout the weeks, or you can make the casserole and eat it for the whole week. You can even freeze individual servings and microwave it when needed. You want your diet to work around your life, not change your life to work around your diet. Too many huge changes at one time can lead to failure. So, find what meals work for you and stick to it, for instance, if you are more likely to hit the snooze button on your alarm and find yourself rushing, setting aside time to cook an elaborate breakfast, might not be feasible. If that is the case, the casserole or the muffins would be best for you.

Chapter 4: Ketogenic Lunches

When it comes to ketogenic friendly foods, it is usually best if you prepare them at home so you know exactly what you're eating. If you have a tendency to go out to lunch when you are at work, bringing it might seem strange in the beginning. However, it is easier than trying to find ketogenic friendly foods on a menu that does not usually have them specifically listed. Going out to eat can be frustrating because you will need to ask the server so many different questions about ingredients. Until you are more comfortable and confident with your diet, it is a good idea to bring your lunch with you, just to ensure that you remain in ketosis.

Just like with the breakfasts, you can make your lunches daily if you choose, or you can prep things a head of time. Some people prefer to only make lunches that can frozen in individual servings so all they have to do is thrown the Tupperware into their lunchbox and be on their way. Others prefer to prepare their lunch night before or their morning of work, depending on time and what they are in the mood for. The following recipes are all easy and quick, and fit well with the mix and match three week plan.

Mixed Green Salad

3 tablespoons roasted pine nuts
2 tablespoons shaved parmesan
2 ounces of mixed greens
2 slices of bacon
Salt and pepper to taste
Ketogenic friendly dressing of your choice, read the label carefully

1. Cook the bacon until it is crispy, you can do this the oven or in a pan, it is up to you. Some people prefer to burn the edges just a bit to add bitter notes to the salad, this complements vinaigrette dressings especially well.

2. Put your portioned greens into a container that has a lid with some extra room, this is for shaking purposes, so keep that in mind when choosing.
3. Crumble the bacon into the greens and toss in the rest of the ingredients including the dressing. Put the lid on the top and shake the container until the dressing coats the greens evenly.

If you are taking this with you to work, wait until you get to work to combine the ingredients. You can keep them separate in reusable bags or in small containers. This helps to keep the salad from getting soggy.

Pigs in a Keto Blanket

37 small sausages, read the label carefully
1 egg
1.5 ounces of cream cheese
8 ounces of cheddar cheese
¾ almond flour
1 tablespoon psyllium husk powder, or coconut flour
Salt and pepper to taste

1. Combine all the dry ingredients in a large bowl.
2. Melt the cheddar cheese in 20 second intervals in the microwave, stir carefully to ensure it is melting evenly. It is done when it is completely melted and slightly bubbling on the outside.
3. Mix together all the ingredients while the cheddar is still hot, this will be your dough.
4. Spread the dough out in a flat and even sheet, make sure it is not too thick, you have 37 sausages to cover after all.
5. Preheat your oven to 400F and put the dough in the refrigerator for 15 to 20 minutes to let it harden up a bit.
6. Once it is cold, slice the dough into strips, a pizza cutter is perfect for this, and wrap them around the sausages. Put them in the oven and bake them for 13 to 15 minutes, before you remove them, broil them for an additional one or two minutes.

These make a great lunch because they can be reheated once you get to work. You can eat them with a sugar-free ketchup or mustard if you choose. In addition to making a convenient lunch, these also make the perfect snack to bring to a party. When you go to gatherings or parties you might find that there is a lack of ketogenic snacks. Unless otherwise specified, it is safe to assume that you might be faced with a table full of foods you can't eat. The easy solution is to bring your own, these are perfect for that.

Tuna Melt Balls with Avocado

10 ounce canned tuna, drained
1 avocado
1/3 cup almond flour
¼ cup mayonnaise, read the label to check for added sugars
¼ cup parmesan cheese
¼ teaspoon onion powder
½ teaspoon garlic powder
Salt and pepper to taste
½ coconut oil for frying, approximately a ¼ cup will be absorbed

1. Drain the tuna and put it a bowl that is large enough to hold all of the ingredients.
2. Add the parmesan cheese, spices, and mayonnaise to the tuna and mix it together until evenly coated.
3. Slice your avocado in half and carefully take out the pit, cube the inside. If you have a way that you prefer to cut avocados, feel free to do what makes you comfortable, just make sure the pieces are in small cubes.
4. Add the avocado in with the rest of the mixture, but fold it in slowly, try not to mash it too much, you want pieces to remain.
5. Roll the mixture into balls, about the size of traditional meat balls. Then roll them in the almond flour, make sure they are evenly coated.
6. Put the coconut oil in a pan on medium heat, when it is hot add the tuna balls and fry them until they are brown and crisp on the

outside. Make sure you are turning them to ensure each side is cooked properly.

7. Now, simply remove from the pan and serve.

These are a great ketogenic version of a tuna melt, you get the creamy center and the added crunch of the outside. Granted, they are not going to be as crunchy when they are reheated, but they are still delicious and easy to take to work with you.

Pizza Frittata

9 ounce bag frozen spinach
12 eggs
1 ounce pepperoni
1 teaspoon minced garlic
5 ounce mozzarella cheese
½ cup parmesan cheese
½ cup fresh ricotta cheese
4 tablespoons olive oil
¼ teaspoon nutmeg
Salt and pepper to taste
Iron skillet or glass container

1. Microwave the frozen spinach for three to four minutes, you don't want to be hot, just defrosted. Then squeeze the spinach with your hands to remove as much water as you can and then set it aside.
2. Preheat your oven to 375F and while it is getting hot, mix together the olive oil, eggs, and spices. Stir or whisk this together until everything is combined.
3. Break the spinach up into small pieces and toss it in the mixture. Next, add the parmesan and ricotta cheeses and mix everything together until it is well combined.
4. Pour your mixture into the skillet and then cover with the mozzarella, place the pepperoni on top just like you would a traditional pizza.

5. Put in the oven and bake for 30 minutes if you are using the cast iron skillet, add an additional 10 to 15 minutes if it is glass. You might need to adjust the baking time depending on the thickness of the frittata, but you will know when it is done when it is slightly browned and firm.
6. Then, just slice and serve.

This a perfect lunch to make at the beginning of the week, that will provide enough servings to last the entire week. It is easy to bring to work and once you are there, you can simply heat it up.

Chicken and BBQ Soup

Base
2 teaspoons chili seasoning
3 chicken thighs
1 ½ cups chicken broth
2 tablespoons of olive oil or chicken fat
1 ½ cups of beef broth
Salt and pepper to taste

Sauce
1 tablespoon hot sauce
¼ cup reduced sugar ketchup
2 tablespoons Dijon mustard
¼ cup tomato paste
1 teaspoon Worcestershire sauce
2 1.2 teaspoon liquid smoke
1 tablespoon soy sauce
1 teaspoon onion powder
1 teaspoon red chili flakes
1 teaspoon chili powder
1 teaspoon cumin
¼ cup butter
1 ½ teaspoons garlic powder
Crock pot or slow cooker

1. Preheat the oven to 400F and remove the bones from the chicken thighs and keep the bones. Season the chicken with some of the chili seasoning and put on a baking tray that is lined with foil.

2. Place the chicken in the oven and bake for 50 minutes.

3. While the chicken is in the oven, grab a pot and add the chicken fat or olive oil, heat this on medium high heat and when it is hot put the chicken bones into the oil and cook them for five minutes. Next, add the broth and season with salt and pepper to taste.

4. When the chicken is done baking, take them out and remove the skins and set aside. Pour the fat from the baked chicken into the broth, stirring occasionally.

5. Now you are going to BBQ sauce by combining all of the ingredients listed above. Then add it to the large pot and stir everything together. Let the mixture simmer for about 20 to 30 minutes.

6. After it has had time to simmer, use an immersion blender, this will emulsify the liquids and fats together. Shred the chicken and put it in the soup, you can also add bell pepper or spring onions during this step if you choose to and simmer for another 10 to 20 minutes.

7. After it has had time to thicken up, you can now serve it up. You can garnish it with a little cheddar cheese, onions, or some diced up green peppers. The crispy chicken you set aside should also be served on the side as well, it makes a great texture addition to the meal.

This is a great lunch option because you can put individual servings in plastic containers and either refrigerate or freeze them for later use. Then when you need a quick lunch on the go, grab the container, throw it your lunch box and be on your way. If that works better for you, than you should really consider utilizing more recipes like these.

Grilled Cheese Keto Style

'Bread'

2 tablespoons almond flour
2 eggs
1 ½ tablespoons psyllium husk powder
2 tablespoons soft butter
½ teaspoon baking powder

Extras

1 tablespoon butter, soft
2 ounces of white or traditional cheddar

1. Combine the butter, almond flour, baking powder, and psyllium husk in a small bowl.
2. Stir this mixture together as much as you can, it will take the form of a very thick dough.
3. Add the 2 eggs and mix it together, you want your dough to be thick, so it seems too thin, keep mixing it together, as this will help thicken it up. This can take a full minute or more so be patient.
4. Scoop half the dough out into a square container roughly the size of a slice of bread, or the bottom a bowl to create bun, try to make sure it is spread evenly. You can also use a slightly larger container and cut in half later, if that is what you choose to do, use all the batter. Microwave this for a 90 to 100 seconds. Some might take a little longer to cook thoroughly so check it and it if it still too soft, microwave it for a little longer.
5. Gently remove it from the container by turning it upside down and tapping on the bottom of the container. If you used all of your batter you can cut it in half, if you need to repeat the process to create the other slice of bread, then do so.
6. Place the cheese in between the slices of bread.

7. In a pan set on medium heat add the butter and when it is hot add the sandwich. The bread will absorb the butter creating that delicious crisp, once it is golden brown, flip and cook the other side until golden brown.

8. Lastly, it is time to eat! A small side salad makes the perfect addition to this gooey, cheesy dish.

This is a great comfort food and probably one of the things that you will find yourself craving rather frequently. Again, just because you are on the ketogenic diet does not mean you have to give up everything you love, you just need to learn to make it in new and different ways that won't compromise ketosis.

Remember, this is a mix and match meal plan, you do not have to eat all the meals, but do try to keep an open mind. There is no lack of variety when it comes to the ketogenic diet, as a matter of fact, you can still have many of the foods you crave, they will just have a bit of a twist added to them. Whether or not you choose to make your lunches for the whole week or that day is up to you, but you do have the option. Keep in mind, this will get much easier the more you practice. In the beginning, the key is planning and sticking to it. If you need to create a weekly menu to keep you on track, then do it, there is nothing wrong with it. This is your diet and you have the right to do what works for you.

Chapter 5: Ketogenic Dinners

When it comes to dinners you can be a bit more creative because there isn't typically the need to grab it and go. Most people have more time to cook a dinner and not have to worry about making enough for a full week or whether or not it will travel well. Just like with the other recipes, you are going to choose your ingredients and keep track of the net carbohydrates you are consuming and since this is the last meal of the day, you will have a good idea of how many net carbohydrates you have let to devote to your dinner.

If you have a big dinner planned that you will use up more of your net carbohydrates than usual, make sure to limit your other meals and snacks throughout the day to give yourself the surplus you need for the special dinner. Try not to make this a habit, but everyone has some type of special occasion that requires a more elaborate dinner and this is still possible on the ketogenic diet, it just takes some extra planning. Here is a list of dinner recipes that are perfect for a ketogenic beginner.

Chicken with Creamy Greens

1 cup chicken stock
1 pound boneless chicken thighs, with skin still on
1 cup cream
2 cups dark leafy greens
2 tablespoons coconut oil
2 tablespoons coconut flour
2 tablespoons melted butter
1 teaspoon Italian herbs
Salt and pepper to taste

1. In a skillet set on medium high heat add the coconut oil. While this is getting hot, season the chicken with the salt and pepper, make sure to do both sides. When the oil is hot enough, brown the chicken on both sides

2. Continue to fry the chicken until it is crispy and cooked thoroughly. When you are cooking the chicken, you should also start making your sauce.

3. In a sauce pan melt the butter, when it stops sizzling, this means do not let it get brown, only melted, add the coconut flour and begin to whisk it together. Continue to whisk until it forms a thick paste.

4. Add the cream and increase the heat to bring it to a boil, continue to whisk. It will begin to thicken again and when it does, add the Italian herbs.

5. When your chicken is done frying, remove them from the stove and take out the thighs and set them aside.

6. Add the chicken stock into the skillet that just had the chicken in it and deglaze the skillet, slowly add the cream sauce and whisk. Slowly stir the greens into the sauce so they become evenly coated with the sauce.

7. Place the chicken on top of the greens and remove from the stove. You can now serve the meal, when dividing, it makes four servings.

Walnut Crusted Salmon

2 tablespoons sugar-free maple syrup
2, 3 ounce salmon fillets
½ cup walnuts
1 tablespoon olive oil
¼ teaspoon dill
½ tablespoon Dijon mustard
Salt and pepper to taste

1. Preheat oven to 350F.

2. Put all the walnuts in a food processor with the spices, mustard, and maple syrup. Blend this together until the consistency is very paste like.

3. In a skillet or pan heat up the olive oil until it is very hot, while this is happening dry both sides of the salmon, make sure to a

do a good job. When the pan is very hot place the salmon in the pan skin down. Allow it to sear for three minutes.

4. While it searing, spoon the walnut mixture onto the fillets.
5. When they have finished being seared, place them on a pan or foil and place them in the oven to bake for around 8 minutes.
6. This is typically served on a bed of fresh spinach, but if you prefer other leafy greens, the choice is yours.

This is a quick and delicious dinner that will leave you feeling satisfied.

Crispy Baked Chicken Wings

3 pounds of wings
1 teaspoon baking soda
¼ cup of butter
1 tablespoon salt
2 teaspoons of baking powder

1. In a large plastic bag, dump in the salt, baking powder, baking soda, and all of the chicken wings.
2. Then shake the bag until all of the wings are coated in the mixture, try to make sure it is as even as possible.
3. Put all of the wings on a wire rack and leave in the refrigerator overnight, this will help them dry out which breaks the peptide bonds in the proteins.
4. The next day, preheat your oven to 450F and place the wings in the top middle rack, bake these for 20 minutes.
5. After the first 20 minutes, flip each wing over and bake for an additional 15 minutes or until they are as crispy as you like the,
6. To make a quick buffalo sauce mix together butter and hot sauce and toss them in this to make ketogenic buffalo wings. Enjoy!

This is a great dinner for when you have been watching your friends get their favorite wings from the local spot. When the craving for this type of comfort food hits you, now you can also enjoy them as well.

Stuffed Poblanos

1 tablespoon bacon fat
1 pound ground pork
½ onion
4 poblano peppers
7 baby bella mushrooms
1 teaspoon cumin
1 vine tomato
1 teaspoon chili powder
¼ cup chopped cilantro
Salt and pepper to taste

1. Rinse and prep all the vegetables, you want to mince garlic, slice the mushrooms and onions, and dice the tomatoes. If your cilantro is not already chopped, do this as well.
2. Set your oven to broil, while this is heating up, place the poblanos on a cookie sheet and put them in the oven when it is hot. Broil them for around 8 to 10 minutes, make sure to move them around every two minutes, you want consistent marks over the entire pepper. Then preheat your oven to 350F.
3. Using a paper towel or gloves to cover your fingers, carefully pull the skin from the peppers. Also, set the skin aside.
4. In a pan that is set on medium high-heat, begin to cook the pork, this is also where you add the bacon fat. Season with salt and pepper, but do not taste it until it has cooked all the way.
5. When it is browned you may now add the chili powder and cumin.
6. In the pan, slide all of the pork to one side and add the garlic and onions to the other side, you want them to be softened.
7. When those have softened add the mushrooms and mix all of it together, add more salt and pepper to suit your palate.

8. When the mixture starts to dry out a little add the tomatoes and cilantro.
9. Make a slice in the poblano pepper from the bottom to the stem and use a spoon or your fingers to remove the seeds. The seeds are spicy, so if you are sensitive to spicy foods, be sure to remove all of them.
10. Carefully fill each pepper with the pork mixture and bake them for around 8 to 10 minutes.
11. Remove them from the oven and they are now ready to serve!

These make a unique and fun dinner for what you are craving something simple and spicy. They will probably become a staple in your new diet if you enjoy spicier foods.

Coconut Shrimp

Shrimp

Egg whites from two eggs
1 pound shrimp, deveined and peeled
2 tablespoons coconut flour
1 cup coconut flakes, unsweetened

Chili Sauce

1 ½ tablespoon rice wine vinegar
1 diced red chili
½ cup apricot preserves, sugar-free
¼ red pepper flakes
1 tablespoon lime juice

1. If you are using frozen shrimp, make sure you thaw them out first, otherwise, if you bought them fresh peel and devein them if needed. Preheat your oven to 375F.

2. Put the egg whites in a bowl and beat them until soft peaks begin to form, this works best using a hand mixer, or if you are in a pinch, one beater inside a blender also works too.
3. In one bowl put the coconut flakes, in another the coconut flour. Take this time to also grease a cookie sheet.
4. Dip the shrimp in the flour, then dip them in the egg whites, and lastly, the flakes. Arrange them on the greased cookie sheet and bake them for about 15 minutes, make sure to flip them and broil for 3 to 5 more minutes.
5. To make the sauce simply add all the ingredients into a bowl mix them together. You might have some left over sauce, but it also goes well with chicken!

These are a great alternative to chicken nuggets or fried shrimp.

Dinners are generally the most fun part of ketogenic cooking because you can really experiment to find what pleases your palate. There are so many different recipes out there already, and you can tweak them so they work for your specific diet needs. Just remember, it might be overwhelming and difficult in the beginning, but you can do it. Just don't give up, let your body adjust and celebrate the small victories like the first pound lost or the first time you didn't have a carb craving all day. This will make the diet more fun and will help keep you motivated.

Chapter 6: Ketogenic Snacks

You are not locked in to only eating three meals a day with no snacking in between. Actually, you can graze a bit throughout the day if that works for you. However, not all snacks are created equal and some are much better than others. Just make sure not to let snacking get out of hand to the point that you are knocked out of ketosis because of it. Don't forget to add in the net carbohydrates from any of the snacks you have eaten throughout the day too, you want an authentic carbohydrate count and this will help make sure it is correct.

The best kind of snacks are the ones that you do not have to spend time preparing, and even though the ketogenic diet is best when you cook at home, there are some things that you can still just grab.

Ketogenic Snacks

Beef, pork, or chicken jerky

String Cheese

Seeds, sunflower, pumpkin, and chia

Pork rinds, just make sure to read the label, you can even dip them in ketogenic friendly dips such as Ranch or Bleu Cheese dressings.

Nut Butters, almond, coconut, and sunflower

Sugar-free jello

Cocoa nibs, this is the perfect alternative to a chocolate bar

In the beginning you might find yourself losing energy or getting hungry at weird times of the day, remember your body is learning to run on something new. So, this is completely normal. These snacks are easy to keep on hand and require no preparation. Just make sure to add them into your daily carbohydrate intake and they should help you during your transition to a low carbohydrate lifestyle.

It probably seems like this diet is overwhelming, but as soon as you get through the first couple of weeks and see the results, you will understand how beneficial it can really be. It will be difficult in the beginning, but you can and should stick it out. You will be proud of yourself in the end. So many people just like you have lost weight and enjoyed healthier lifestyles because of this diet. You don't want to let them reap all the benefits. So, don't let you, hold you back. The secret is finding what works for you and sticking to it, everyone works at their own pace and you are no exception. No matter how badly you might want to compare yourself to others, don't do it. Let your body go at the pace it is meant to, you will learn to know when it is okay to push yourself and when you have truly met your limits, but you won't know either of these until you dedicate yourself and actually try.

PART 2

Chapter 1: Keto Basics

In the introduction we briefly discussed the meaning and theory behind ketogenic dieting. Here we will delve further into the science behind the method and how it can boost your metabolism and detox your body in 10 days.

Benefits of Increased Metabolism

One of the best ways to learn the meaning of a scientific term is to break it down to its roots. When we break down ketogenic we see it is comprised of two words: keto and genic. Ketones are fat-based molecules that the body breaks down when it is using fat as its energy source. When used as a suffix, "genic" means "causing, forming, or producing". So, we put these terms together and we have "ketogenic", or simply put, "causing fat burn". Ergo, the theory behind ketogenic dieting is: when a person reduces the amount of sugar and carbohydrates they consume, the body will begin to breakdown fat it already has in stores all over the body. When your body is cashing in on these stores, it is in a ketogenic state, or "ketosis". When your body consumes food, it naturally seeks carbohydrates for the purpose of breaking them down and using them as fuel. Adversely, a ketogenic cleanse trains your body to use fats for energy instead. This is achieved by lowering the amount of ingested carbohydrates and increasing the amount of ingested fats, which in turn boosts your metabolism.

Only recently has a low carb- high fat diet plan emerged into the public eye. It is a sharp contrast to the traditional dieting style that emphasizes calorie counting. For many years it was over looked that crash diets neglect the most important aspect of dieting: food is fuel. A diet is not meant be treated as a once a year go to method in order to shed holiday weight in January. Rather, a diet is a lifestyle; it is a consistent pattern of how an individual fuels their body. A ten day ketogenic cleanse is the perfect way to begin forming healthy eating habits that overtime become second nature. If you are tired of losing weight just to gain it all back, never fear. We firmly believe that you can accomplish anything you put your mind to, including living a healthy life! You, like hundreds of others, can successfully accomplish a ketogenic cleanse and change the way you see health, fitness, and life along the way. So let's hit the books and get that metabolism working!

Benefits of Cleansing

In addition to increased metabolism and fat loss, ketogenic cleansing allows your body naturally rid itself of harmful toxins and wasteful substances. In today's modern world, food is overrun and polluted by genetically modified hormones, artificial flavors and coloring, and copious amounts of unnecessary sugars. Ketogenic cleansing eliminates breads, grains, and many other foods that are most affected by today's modern industrialization. Due to the high amount of naturally occurring foods used in a ketogenic cleanse, the body is able to obtain many vitamins and minerals that are not prevalent in a high carb diet. When the body is consuming sufficient amounts of necessary vitamins and minerals, it is able to heal itself and maintain a healthy immune system. Cleansing your body is one of the best ways to achieve, and maintain, pristine health.

Chapter 2: Meal Plan Madness

One of the best ways to stay motivated, when dieting, is to find a meal plan that is easy to follow and easy on the budget. Ketogenic meals are designed to be filling while keeping within the perimeters of low-carb, high-fat guidelines. Ideally you want to aim for 70% fats, 25% protein, and 5% carbohydrates in your diet. As long as the materials you use to build your meals are low in carbs and high in fats, feel free to experiment and find what is right for you. Each and every one of us is different and that's okay. After all, this meal plan is for YOU!

Below is a ten day meal plan, designed with a busy schedule in mind, which will not break the bank! All of these meals can be prepared in 30 minutes or less, and many of them are much quicker than that! There is also a list of ingredients for each meal located in the recipe chapter so you can go to the grocery store knowing exactly what you need!

	Breakfast	Lunch	Dinner
Day 1	California Chicken Omelet • Fat: 32 grams • 10 minutes to prepare • Protein: 25 grams • 10 minutes of cooking • Net carbs: 4 grams	Cobb Salad • Fat: 48 grams • 10 minutes to prepare • Protein: 43 grams • 0 minutes of cooking • Net carbs: 3 grams	Chicken Peanut Pad Thai • Fat: 12 grams • 15 minutes to prepare • Protein: 30 grams • 15 minutes of cooking • Net carbs: 2 grams
Day 2	Easy Blender Pancakes • Fat: 29 grams • 5 minutes to prepare • Protein: 41 grams • 10 minutes of cooking	Sardine Stuffed Avocados • Fat: 29 grams • 10 minutes to prepare • Protein: 27 grams	Chipotle Fish Tacos • Fat: 20 grams • 5 minutes to prepare • Protein: 24 grams

	• Net carbs: 4 grams	• 0 minutes of cooking • Net Carbs: 5 grams	• 15 minutes of cooking • Net carbs: 5 grams
Day 3	**Steak and Eggs** • Fat: 36 grams • 10 minutes to prepare • Protein: 47 grams • 5 minutes of cooking • Net carbs: 3 grams	**Low-Carb Smoothie Bowl** • Fat 35 grams • 5 minutes to prepare • Protein: 20 grams • 0 minutes of cooking • Net carbs: 5 grams	**Avocado Lime Salmon** • Fat: 27 grams • 20 minutes to prepare • Protein: 37 grams • 10 minutes of cooking • Net carbs: 5 grams
KEEP IT UP!!!	During the course of your plan, especially around days 3 and 4, you may begin to feel like you don't have it in you. You may have thoughts telling you that you cannot last for ten days on this type pf cleanse. Do not allow feelings of discouragement bother you because, guess what? We all feel that way sometimes! A ketogenic diet causes your body to process energy like it never has before. Keep pressing on! Your body will thank you and so will you!		
Day 4	**Low-Carb Smoothie Bowl** • Fat: 35 grams • 5 minutes to prepare • Protein: 35 grams • 0 minutes of cooking • Net carbs: 4 grams	**Pesto Chicken Salad** • Fat: 27 grams • 5 minutes to prepare • Protein: 27 grams • 10 minutes of cooking • Net carbs: 3 grams	**Siracha Lime Flank Steak** • Fat: 32 grams • 5 minutes to prepare • Protein: 48 grams • 10 minutes of cooking • Net Carbs: 5 grams
Day 5	**Feta and Pesto Omelet** • Fat: 46 grams • 5 minutes of preparation	**Roasted Brussel Sprouts** • Fat: 21 grams • 5 minutes to prepare	**Low carb Sesame Chicken** • Fat: 36 grams • 15 minutes to prepare

	<ul><li>Protein: 30 grams</li><li>5 minutes of cooking</li><li>Net carbs: 2.5 grams</li></ul>	<ul><li>Protein: 21 grams</li><li>30 minutes of cooking</li><li>Net carbs: 4 grams</li></ul>	<ul><li>Protein: 41 grams</li><li>15 minutes of cooking</li><li>Net carbs: 4 grams</li></ul>
Day 6	**Raspberry Cream Crepes**<ul><li>Fat: 40 grams</li><li>5 minutes of preparation</li><li>Net carbs: 8 grams</li><li>15 minutes of cooking</li><li>Protein 15 grams</li></ul>	**Shakshuka**<ul><li>Fat: 34 grams</li><li>Protein 35 grams</li><li>Net carbs: 4 grams</li><li>10 minutes of preparation</li><li>10 minutes of cooking</li></ul>	**Sausage in a Pan**<ul><li>Fat: 38 grams</li><li>10 minutes of preparation</li><li>Protein: 30 grams</li><li>25 minutes of cooking</li><li>Net Carbs: 4 grams</li></ul>
Day 7	**Green Monster Smoothie**<ul><li>Fat: 25 grams</li><li>5 minutes of preparation</li><li>Protein: 30 grams</li><li>0 minutes of cooking</li><li>Net Carbs: 3 grams</li></ul>	**Tuna Tartare**<ul><li>Fat: 24 grams</li><li>15 minutes of preparation</li><li>Protein: 56 grams</li><li>0 minutes of cooking</li><li>Net Carbs: 4 grams</li></ul>	**Pesto Chicken Salad**<ul><li>Fat: 27 grams</li><li>5 minutes of preparation</li><li>Protein: 27 grams</li><li>10 minutes of cooking</li><li>Net carbs: 3 grams</li></ul>
ALMOST THERE!!	By now, you can be certain you are seeing physical results such as reduced body fat and more energy! You are doing a fantastic job and you only have three days left! Keep up the good work, you owe it to yourself.		
Day 8	**Shakshuka**<ul><li>Fat: 34 grams</li><li>10 minutes of preparation</li><li>Protein 35 grams</li><li>10 minutes of cooking</li><li>Net carbs: 4 grams</li></ul>	**Grilled Halloumi Salad**<ul><li>Fat: 47 grams</li><li>15 minutes of preparation</li><li>Protein: 21 grams</li></ul>	**Keto Quarter Pounder**<ul><li>Fat: 34 grams</li><li>10 minutes of preparation</li><li>Protein: 25 grams</li></ul>

		• 0 minutes of cooking • Net carbs: 2 grams	• 8 minutes of cooking • Net carbs: 4 •
Day 9	**Easy Blender Pancakes** • Fat: 29 grams • 5 minutes of preparation • Protein: 41 grams • 10 minutes of cooking • Net carbs: 4 grams	**Broccoli Bacon Salad** • Fat: 31 grams • 15 minutes of preparation • Protein: 10 grams • 6 minutes of cooking • Net carbs: 5 grams	**Sardine Stuffed Avocados** • Fat: 29 grams • 10 minutes to prepare • Protein: 27 grams • 0 minutes to cook • Net Carbs: 5 grams
Day 10	**California Chicken Omelet** • Fat 32 grams • 10 minutes to prepare • Protein 25 grams • 10 minutes of cooking • Net carb: 3 grams	**Shrimp Scampi** • Fat: 21 grams • 5 minutes to prepare • Protein: 21 grams • 30 minutes of cooking • Net carbs: 4 grams	**Tuna Tartare** • Fat: 36 grams • 15 minutes to prepare • Protein: 41 grams • 15 minutes of cooking • Net carbs: 4 grams
YOU DID IT!!	Congratulations! You have successfully completed a 10 day ketogenic cleanse. By now your body has adjusted to its new source of energy, expelled dozens of harmful toxins, and replenished itself with many vitamins and minerals it may have been lacking. Way to go on a job well done!		

Chapter 3: Breakfast Is For Champions

Breakfast is by far the most important meal of the day for one reason: it set the tone for the rest of your day. In order to hit the ground running, it is vital that one starts each day with foods that fuel an energetic and productive day. This chapter contains ten ketogenic breakfast ides that will have you burning fat and conquering your day like you never imagined.

1. California Chicken Omelet

- This recipe requires 10 minutes of preparation, 10 minutes of cooking time and serves 1
- Net carbs: 4 grams
- Protein: 25 grams
- Fat : 32 grams

What you will need:

- Mayo (1 tablespoon)
- Mustard (1 teaspoon)
- Campari tomato
- Eggs (2 large beaten)
- Avocado (one fourth, sliced)
- Bacon (2 slices cooked and chopped)
- Deli chicken (1 ounce)

What to do:

1. Place a skillet on the stove over a burner set to a medium heat and let it warm before adding in the eggs and seasoning as needed.
2. Once eggs are cooked about halfway through, add bacon, chicken, avocado, tomato, mayo, and mustard on one side of the eggs.
3. Fold the omelet onto its self, cover and cook for 5 additional minutes.
4. Once eggs are fully cooked and all ingredients are warm, through the center, your omelet is ready.
5. Bon apatite!

2. Steak and Eggs with Avocado

- This recipe requires 10 minutes of preparation, 5 minutes of cooking time and serves 1
- Net Carbs: 3 grams
- Protein: 44 grams
- Fat: 36 grams

What you will need:

- Salt and pepper
- Avocado (one fourth, sliced)
- Sirloin steak (4 ounce)
- Eggs (3 large)
- Butter (1 tablespoon)

What to do:

1. Melt the tablespoon of butter in a pan and fry all 3 eggs to desired doneness. Season the eggs with salt and pepper.
2. In a different pan, cook the sirloin steak to your preferred taste and slice it into thin strips. Season the steak with salt and pepper.
3. Sever your prepared steak and eggs with slices of avocado.
4. Enjoy!

3. Pancakes an a Blender

- This recipe requires 5 minutes of preparation, 10 minutes of cooking time and serves 1
- Net Carbs: 4 grams
- Protein: 41 grams
- Fat: 29 grams

What you will need:

- Whey protein powder (1 scoop)
- Eggs (2 large)
- Cream cheese (2 ounces)
- Just a pinch of cinnamon and a pinch of salt

What to do:

1. Combine cream cheese, eggs, protein powder, cinnamon, and salt into a blender. Blend for 10 seconds and let stand.
2. While letting batter stand, warm a skillet over medium heat.
3. Pour about ¼ of the batter onto warmed skillet and let cook. When bubbles begin to emerge on the surface, flip the pancake.
4. Once flipped, cook for 15 seconds. Repeat until remainder of the batter is used up.
5. Top with butter and/ or sugar- free maple syrup and you are all set!
6. Chow time!

4. Low Carb Smoothe Bowl

- Net Carbs: 4 grams
- Protein: 35 grams
- Fat: 35 grams
- Takes 5 minutes to prepare and serves 1.

What you will need:

- Spinach (1 cup)
- Almond milk (half a cup)
- Coconut oil (1 tablespoon)
- Low carb protein powder (1 scoop)
- Ice cubes (2 cubes)
- Whipping cream (2 T)
- Optional toppings can include: raspberries, walnuts, shredded coconut, or chia seeds

What to do:

1. Place spinach in blender. Add almond milk, cream, coconut oil, and ice. Blend until thoroughly and evenly combined.
2. Pour into bowl.
3. Top with toppings or stir lightly into smoothie.
4. Treat yourself!

5. Feta and Pesto Omelet

- This recipe requires 5 minutes of preparation, 5 minutes of cooking time and serves 1
- Net Carbs: 2.5 grams
- Protein: 30 grams
- Fat: 46 grams

What you will need:

- Butter (1 tablespoon)
- Eggs (3 large)
- Heavy cream (1 tablespoon)
- Feta cheese (1 ounce)
- Basil pesto (1 teaspoon)
- Tomatoes (optional)

What to do:

1. Heat pan and melt butter.
2. Beat eggs together with heavy whipping cream (will give eggs a fluffy consistency once cooked).
3. Pour eggs in pan and cook until almost done, add feta and pesto to on half of eggs.
4. Fold omelet and cook for an additional 4-5 minutes.
5. Top with feta and tomatoes, and eat up!

6. Crepes with Cream and Raspberries

- This recipe requires 5 minutes of preparation, 15 minutes of cooking time and serves 2
- Net Carbs: 8 grams
- Protein: 15 grams
- Fat: 40 grams

What you will need:

- Raspberries (3 ounces, fresh or frozen)
- Whole Milk Ricotta (half a cup and 2 tablespoons)
- Erythritol (2 tablespoons)
- Eggs (2 large)
- Cream Cheese (2 ounces)
- Pinch of salt
- Dash of Cinnamon
- Whipped cream and sugar- free maple syrup to go on top

What to do:

1. In a blender, blend cream cheese, eggs, erythritol, salt, and cinnamon for about 20 seconds, or until there are no lumps of cream cheese.
2. Place a pan on a burner turned to a medium heat before coating in cooking spray. Add 20 percent of your batter to the pan in a thin layer. Cook crepe until the underside becomes slightly darkened. Carefully flip the crepe and let the reverse side cook for about 15 seconds.
3. Repeat step 3 until all batter is used.
4. Without stacking the crepes, allow them to cool for a few minutes.
5. After the crepes have cool, place about 2 tablespoons of ricotta cheese in the center of each crepe.
6. Throw in a couple of raspberries and fold the side to the middle.
7. Top those off with some whipped cream and sugar- free maple syrup and…
8. Viola! You're a true chef! Indulge in your creation!

7. Green Monster Smoothie

- This recipe requires 10 minutes of preparation, 0 minutes of cooking time and serves 1
- Net Carbs: 4 grams
- Protein: 30 grams
- Fat: 25 grams

What you will need:

- Almond milk (one and a half cups)
- Spinach (one eighth of a cup)
- Cucumber (fourth of a cup)
- Celery (fourth of a cup)
- Avocado (fourth of a cup)
- Coconut oil (1 tablespoon)
- Stevia (liquid, 10 drops)
- Whey Protein Powder (1 scoop)

What to do:

1. In a blender, blend almond milk and spinach for a few pulses.
2. Add remaining ingredients and blend until thoroughly combined.
3. Add optional matcha powder, if desired, and enjoy!

Chapter 4: Lunch Crunch

Eating a healthy lunch when you are limited on time due to, work, school, or taking care of your kids can be a tumultuous task. Thankfully, we have compiled a list of eight quick and easy recipes to accompany the ten day meal plan laid out in chapter 2! Many find it advantageous, especially if you work throughout the week, to prepare you meals ahead of time. Thankfully, these lunch recipes are also easy to pack and take on the go!

1. Off The Cobb Salad

- Net carbs: 3 grams
- Protein: 43 grams
- Fat: 48 grams
- Takes 10 minutes to prepare and serves 1.

What you will need:

- Spinach (1 cup)
- Egg (1, hard-boiled)
- Bacon (2 strips)
- Chicken breast (2 ounces)
- Campari tomato (one half of tomato)
- Avocado (one fourth, sliced)
- White vinegar (half of a teaspoon)
- Olive oil (1 tablespoon)

What to do:

1. Cook chicken and bacon completely and cut or slice into small pieces.
2. Chop remaining ingredients into bite size pieces.
3. Place all ingredients, including chicken and bacon, in a bowl, toss ingredients in oil and vinegar.
4. Enjoy!

2. Avocado and Sardines

- Net Carbs: 5 grams
- Protein: 27 grams
- Fat: 52 grams
- Takes 10 minutes to prepare and serves 1.

What you will need:

- Fresh lemon juice (1 tablespoon)
- Spring onion or chives (1 or small bunch)
- Mayonnaise (1 tablespoon)
- Sardines (1 tin, drained)
- Avocado (1 whole, seed removed)
- Turmeric powder (fourth of a teaspoon) or freshly ground turmeric root (1 teaspoon)
- Salt (fourth of a teaspoon)

What to do:

1. Begin by cutting the avocado in half and removing its seed.
2. Scoop out about half the avocado and set aside (shown below).
3. In small bowl, mash drained sardines with fork.
4. Add onion (or chives), turmeric powder, and mayonnaise. Mix well.
5. Add removed avocado to sardine mixture.
6. Add lemon juice and salt.
7. Scoop the mixture into avocado halves.
8. Dig in!

3. Chicken Salad A La Pesto

- This recipe requires 5minutes of preparation, 10 minutes of cooking time and serves 4
- Net Carbs: 3 grams
- Protein: 27 grams
- Fat: 27 grams

What you will need:

- Garlic pesto (2 tablespoons)
- Mayonnaise (fourth of a cup)
- Grape tomatoes (10, halved)
- Avocado (1, cubed)
- Bacon (6 slices, cooked crisp and crumbled)
- Chicken (1 pound, cooked and cubed)
- Romaine lettuce (optional)

What to do:

1. Combine all ingredients in a large mixing bowl.
2. Toss gently to spread mayonnaise and pesto evenly throughout.
3. If desired, wrap in romaine lettuce for a low-carb BLT chicken wrap.
4. Bon apatite!

4. Bacon and Roasted Brussel Sprouts

- This recipe requires 5 minutes of preparation, 30 minutes of cooking time and serves 4
- Net Carbs: 4 grams
- Protein: 15 grams
- Fat: 21 grams

What you will need:

- Bacon (8 strips)
- Olive oil (2 tablespoons)
- Brussel sprouts (1 pound, halved)
- Salt and pepper

What to do:

1. Preheat oven to 375 degrees Fahrenheit.
2. Gently mix Brussel sprouts with olive oil, salt, and pepper.
3. Spread Brussel sprouts evenly onto a greased baking sheet.
4. Bake in oven for 30 minutes. Shake the pan about halfway through to mix the Brussel sprout halves up a bit.
5. While Brussel sprouts are in the oven, fry bacon slices on stovetop.
6. When bacon is fully cooked, let cool and chop it into bite size pieces.
7. Combine bacon and Brussel sprouts in a bowl and you're finished!
8. Feast!!

5. Grilled Halloumi Salad

- Net Carbs: 7 grams
- Protein: 21 grams
- Fat: 47 grams
- Takes 15 minutes to prepare and serves 1.

What you will need:

- Chopped walnuts (half of an ounce)
- Baby arugula (1 handful)
- Grape tomatoes (5)
- Cucumber (1)
- Halloumi cheese (3 ounces)
- Olive oil (1 teaspoon)
- Balsamic vinegar (half of a teaspoon)
- A pinch of salt

What to do:

1. Slice halloumi cheese into slices 1/3 of an in thick.
2. Grill cheese for 3 to 5 minutes, until you see grill lines, on each side.
3. Wash and cut veggies into bite size pieces, place in salad bowl.
4. Add rinsed baby arugula and walnuts to veggies.
5. Toss in olive oil, balsamic vinegar, and salt.
6. Place grilled halloumi on top of veggies and your lunch is ready!
7. Eat those greens and get back to work!

6. Bacon Broccoli Salad

- This recipe requires 15 minutes of preparation, 6 minutes of cooking time and serves 5.
- Net Carbs: 5 grams
- Protein: 10 grams
- Fat: 31 grams

What you will need:

- Sesame oil (half of a teaspoon)
- Erythritol (1 and a half tablespoons) or stevia to taste
- White vinegar (1 tablespoon)
- Mayonnaise (half of a cup)
- Green onion (three fourths of an ounce)
- Bacon (fourth of a pound)
- Broccoli (1 pound, heads and stalks cut and trimmed)

What to do:

1. Cook bacon and crumble into bits.
2. Cut broccoli into bite sized pieces.
3. Slice scallions.
4. Mix mayonnaise, vinegar, erythritol (or stevia), and sesame oil, to make the dressing.
5. Place broccoli and bacon bits in a bowl and toss with dressing.
6. Viola!

7. Tuna Avocado Tartare

- Net Carbs: 4 grams
- Protein: 56 grams
- Fat: 24 grams
- Takes 15 minutes to prepare and serves 2.

What you will need:

- Sesame seed oil (2 tablespoons)
- Sesame seeds (1 teaspoon)
- Cucumbers (2)
- Lime (half of a whole lime)
- Mayonnaise (1 tablespoon)
- Sriracha (1 tablespoon)
- Olive oil (2 tablespoons)
- Jalapeno (one half of whole jalapeno)
- Scallion (3 stalks)
- Avocado (1)
- Tuna steak (1 pound)
- Soy sauce (1 tablespoon)

What to do:

1. Dice tuna and avocado into ¼ inch cubes, place in bowl.
2. Finely chop scallion and jalapeno, add to bowl.
3. Pour olive oil, sesame oil, siracha, soy sauce, mayonnaise, and lime into bowl.
4. Using hands, toss all ingredients to combine evenly. Using a utensil may breakdown avocado, which you want to remain chunky, so it is best to use your hands.
5. Top with sesame seeds and serve with a side of sliced cucumber.
6. There's certainly something fishy about this recipe, but it tastes great! Enjoy!

8. Warm Spinach and Shrimp

- This recipe requires 15 minutes of preparation, 6 minutes of cooking time and serves 5.
- Fat: 24 grams
- Protein: 36 grams
- Net Carbs: 3 grams
- Takes10 minutes to prepare, 5 minutes to cook, and serves 2.

What you will need:

- Spinach (2 handfuls)
- Parmesan (half a tablespoon)
- Heavy cream (1 tablespoon)
- Olive oil (1 tablespoon)
- Butter (2 tablespoons)
- Garlic (3 cloves)
- Onion (one fourth of whole onion)
- Large raw shrimp (about 20)
- Lemon (optional)

What to do:

1. Place peeled shrimp in cold water.
2. Chop onions and garlic into fine pieces.
3. Heat oil, in pan, over medium heat. Cook shrimp in oil until lightly pink (we do not want them fully cooked here). Remove shrimp from oil and set aside.
4. Place chopped onions and garlic into pan, cook until onions are translucent. Add a dash of salt.
5. Add butter, cream, and parmesan cheese. Stir until you have a smooth sauce.
6. Let sauce cook for about 2 minutes so it will thicken slightly.
7. Place shrimp back into pan and cook until done. This should take no longer than 2 or 3 minutes. Be careful not to overcook the shrimp, it will become dry and tough!
8. Remove shrimp and sauce from pan and replace with spinach. Cook spinach VERY briefly
9. Place warmed spinach onto a plate.
10. Pour shrimp and sauce over bed of spinach, squeeze some lemon on top, if you like, and you're ready to chow down!

Chapter 5: Thinner by Dinner

It's the end of the day and you are winding down from a hard day's work. Your body does not require a lot of energy while you sleep; therefore, dinner will typically consist of less fat and more protein.

1. Chicken Pad Thai

- Net Carbs: 7 grams
- Protein: 30 grams
- Fat: 12 grams
- Takes 15 minutes to prepare, 15 minutes to cook, and serves 4.

What you will need:

- Peanuts (1 ounce)
- Lime (1 whole)
- Soy sauce (2 tablespoons)
- Egg (1 large)
- Zucchini (2 large)
- Chicken thighs (16 ounces, boneless and skinless)
- Garlic (2 cloves, minced)
- White onion (1,chopped)
- Olive oil (1 tablespoon)
- Chili flakes (optional)

What to do:

1. Over medium heat, cook olive oil and onion until translucent. Add the garlic and cook about three minutes (until fragrant).
2. Cook chicken in pan for 5 to 7 minutes on each side (until fully cooked). Remove chicken from heat and shred it using a couple of forks.
3. Cut ends off zucchini and cut into thin noodles. Set zucchini noodles aside.
4. Next, scramble the egg in the pan.

5. Once the egg is fully cooked, and the zucchini noodles and cook for about 2 minutes.
6. Add the previously shredded chicken to the pan.
7. Give it some zing with soy sauce, lime juice, peanuts, and chili flakes.
8. Time to eat!

2. Chipotle Style Fish Tacos

- Fat: 20 grams
- Protein: 24 grams
- Net Carbs: 7 grams
- Takes 5 minutes to prepare, 15 minutes to cook, and serves 4.

What you will need:

- Low carb tortillas (4)
- Haddock fillets (1 pound)
- Mayonnaise (2 tablespoons)
- Butter (2 tablespoons)
- Chipotle peppers in adobo sauce (4 ounces)
- Garlic (2 cloves, pressed)
- Jalapeño (1 fresh, chopped)
- Olive oil (2 tablespoons)
- Yellow onion (half of an onion, diced)

What to do:

1. Fry diced onion (until translucent) in olive oil in a high sided pan, over medium- high heat.
2. Reduce heat to medium, add jalapeno and garlic. Cook while stir for another two minutes.
3. Chop the chipotle peppers and add them, along with the adobo sauce, to the pan.
4. Add the butter, mayo, and fish fillets to the pan.
5. Cook the fish fully while breaking up the fillets and stirring the fish into other ingredients.
6. Warm tortillas for 2 minutes on each side.
7. Fill tortillas with fishy goodness and eat up!

3. Salmon with Avocado Lime Sauce

- Net Carbs: 5 grams
- Protein: 37 grams
- Fat: 27 grams
- Takes 20 minutes to prepare, 10 minutes to cook, and serves 2.

What you will need:

- Salmon (two 6 ounce fillets)
- Avocado (1 large)
- Lime (one half of a whole lime)
- Red onion (2 tablespoons, diced)
- Cauliflower (100 grams)

What to do:

1. Chop cauliflower in a blender or food processor then cook it in a lightly oiled pan, while covered, for 8 minutes. This will make the cauliflower rice-like.
2. Next, blend the avocado with squeezed lime juice in the blender or processor until smooth and creamy.
3. Heat some oil in a skillet and cook salmon (skin side down first) for 4 to 5 minute. Flip the fillets and cook for an additional 4 to 5 minutes.
4. Place salmon fillet on a bed of your cauliflower rice and top with some diced red onion.

4. Siracha Lime Steak

- Net Carbs: 5 grams
- Protein: 48 grams
- Fat: 32 grams
- Takes 5 minutes to prepare, 10 minutes to cook, and serves 2.

What you will need:

- Vinegar (1 teaspoon)
- Olive oil (2 tablespoons)
- Lime (1 whole)
- Sriracha (2 tablespoons)
- Flank steak (16 ounce)
- Salt and pepper

What to do:

1. Season steak, liberally, with salt and pepper. Place on baking sheet, lined with foil, and broil in oven for 5 minutes on each side (add another minute or two for a well done steak). Remove from oven, cover, and set aside.
2. Place sriracha in small bowl and squeeze lime into it. Whisk in salt, pepper, and vinegar.
3. Slowly pour in olive oil.
4. Slice steak into thin slices, lather on your sauce, and enjoy!
5. Feel free to pair this recipe with a side of greens such as asparagus or broccoli.

5. Low Carb Sesame Chicken

- Net Carbs: 4 grams
- Protein: 45 grams
- Fat: 36 grams
- Takes 15minutes to prepare, 15 minutes to cook, and serves 2.

What you will need:
- Broccoli (three fourths of a cup, cut bite size)
- Xanthan gum (fourth of a teaspoon)
- Sesame seeds (2 tablespoons)
- Garlic (1 clove)
- Ginger (1 cm cube)
- Vinegar (1 tablespoon)
- Brown sugar alternative (Sukrin Gold is a good one) (2 tablespoons)
- Soy sauce (2 tablespoons)
- Toasted sesame seed oil (2 tablespoons)
- Arrowroot powder or corn starch (1 tablespoon)
- Chicken thighs (1poundcut into bite sized pieces)
- Egg (1 large)
- Salt and pepper
- Chives (optional)

What to do:
1. First we will make the batter by combining the egg with a tablespoon of arrowroot powder (or cornstarch). Whisk well.
2. Place chicken pieces in batter. Be sure to coat all sides of chicken pieces with the batter.
3. Heat one tablespoon of sesame oil, in a large pan. Add chicken pieces to hot oil and fry. Be gentle when flipping the chicken, you want to keep the batter from falling off. It should take about 10 minutes for them to cook fully.
4. Next, make the sesame sauce. In a small bowl, combine soy sauce, brown sugar alternative, vinegar, ginger, garlic, sesame seeds, and the remaining tablespoon of toasted sesame seed oil. Whisk very well.
5. Once the chicken is fully cooked, add broccoli and the sesame sauce to pan and cook for an additional 5 minutes.
6. Spoon desired amount into a bowl, top it off with some chopped chives, and relish in some fine dining at home!

6. Pan 'O Sausage

- Net Carbs: 4 grams
- Protein: 30 grams
- Fat: 38 grams
- Takes 10 minutes to prepare, 25 minutes to cook, and serves 2.

What you will need:

- Basil (half a teaspoon)
- Oregano (half a teaspoon)
- White onion (1 tablespoon)
- Shredded mozzarella (fourth of a cup)
- Parmesan cheese (fourth of a cup)
- Vodka sauce (half a cup)
- Mushrooms (4 ounces)
- Sausage (3 links)
- Salt (fourth of a teaspoon)
- Red pepper (fourth of a teaspoon, ground)

What to do:

1. Preheat oven to 350 degrees Fahrenheit.
2. Heat an iron skillet over medium flame. When skillet is hot, cook sausage links until almost thoroughly cooked.
3. While sausage is cooking, slice mushrooms and onion.
4. When sausage is almost fully cooked, remove links from heat and place mushrooms and onions in skillet to brown.
5. Cut sausage into pieces about ½ inch thick and place pieces in pan.
6. Season skillet contents with oregano, basil, salt, and red pepper.
7. Add vodka sauce and parmesan cheese. Stir everything together.
8. Place skillet in oven for 15 minutes. Sprinkle mozzarella on top a couple minutes before removing dish from oven.
9. Once 15 minutes is up, remove skillet from the oven and let cool for a few minutes.
10. Dinner time!

7. Quarter Pounder Keto Burger

- Net Carbs: 4 grams
- Protein: 25 grams
- Fat: 34 grams
- Takes 10 minutes to prepare, 8 minutes to cook, and serves 2.

What you will need:

- Basil (half a teaspoon)
- Cayenne (fourth a teaspoon)
- Crushed red pepper (half a teaspoon)
- Salt (half a teaspoon)
- Lettuce (2 large leaves)
- Butter (2 tablespoons)
- Egg (1 large)
- Sriracha (1 tablespoon)
- Onion (fourth of whole onion)
- Plum tomato (half of whole tomato)
- Mayo (1 tablespoon)
- Pickled jalapenos (1 tablespoon, sliced)
- Bacon (1 strip)
- Ground beef (half a pound)
- Bacon (1 strip)

What to do:

1. Knead mean for about three minute.
2. Chop bacon, jalapeno, tomato, and onion into fine pieces. (shown below)
3. Knead in mayo, sriracha, egg, and chopped ingredients, and spices into meat.
4. Separate meat into four even pieces and flatten them (not thinly, just press on the tops to create a flat surface). Place a tablespoon of butter on top of two of the meat pieces. Take the pieces that do not have butter of them and set them on top of the buttered

ones (basically creating a butter and meat sandwich). Seal the sides together, concealing the butter within.

5. Throw the patties on the grill (or in a pan) for about 5 minutes on each side. Caramelize some onions if you want too!

6. Prepare large leaves of lettuce by spreading some mayo onto them. Once patties are finished, place them on one half of the lettuce, add your desired burger toppings, and fold the other half over of the lettuce leaf over the patty.

7. Burger time!

PART 3

Chapter 1: A Little Explanation About Whole Food

According to a recent and up-to-date study, a lot of people consume foods that only look like they were prepared with whole wheat flour. This is because of the fact that we are used to white bread, and we ignore some or all of the flour with which it is prepared. For now, we will try to understand what whole products are and why they're good for our body.

Whole food, the real kind

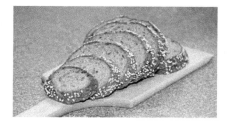

'Whole grain products' refer to products that are composed of whole grains of cereals or derivatives. The whole grains contain all of its component parts: the bran, endosperm, and germ. The process of refining these grains is usually very complicated, and for this reason, their characteristics are often modified to improve their taste or even their color.

Often, without realizing, we buy products because of the color and the word 'whole' on the bag, thinking that they were whole grain but they're not. In fact, if we have a look at the ingredients of that product, we will see that these foods are made mostly from refined flour, and only a small amount of wholemeal flour was used or that bran was simply added. This is because of the fact that, according to American law, it can be called 'whole grain' as long as bran is added to refined flour. So, be sure that before you even buy a product, you should read the ingredients carefully.

The most common whole grain products are whole wheat, wild rice, rye, corn, oats, whole barley, spelt, millet, quinoa, kamut, buckwheat, pearl wheat, amaranth, sorghum, and the flours that are derived from it. As for how much whole grain we should eat, the American Food Safety Authority recommends consuming 25g of fiber a day, and a great way to do this is to incorporate these foods into your diet.

Why whole food is good

The regular consumption of whole foods allows you to take advantage of all their benefits. Whole grains are a great source of beneficial substances for our body. They are rich in dietary fiber, proteins, carbohydrates, vitamins, and mineral salts. There is also a good percentage of antioxidant compounds that are present. Most fibers and vitamin B content are found in the bran. Let's now have a look at the benefits of these foods together:

They prevent hypoglycemic peaks

A negative characteristic of refined flours is that they have high-sugar content that results in the increase of blood sugar and the production of insulin, promoting the onset of Type 2 diabetes. Thanks to the presence of fibers, however, whole foods can induce slow-absorption of sugars to prevent blood sugar peaks.

Whole foods are good for the intestine

When fibers come into contact with water, they increase in volume. This increase in volume stimulates peristalsis, which results in the elimination of waste substances.

Whole foods are good for heart and arteries

Consuming whole food products can help prevent cardiovascular disease because the fibers contained in them reduce the absorption of fats in the blood. This also affects the onset of diseases related to the presence of high levels of LDL cholesterol.

Whole foods are good for dieting

Sugar is addictive and affects our well-being in so many ways. A diet high in fiber helps prevent hunger pangs, even nervous ones, reduces the absorption of sugar and fat. If you decide to consume foods rich in fiber, it is always advisable to drink a lot of water to ensure that feeling of being satiated will stay for a long time. Finally, eating the right food facilitates the correct functioning of the intestine, deflating the stomach and reducing cellulite.

Whole foods are good as a defense

The macronutrients contained in whole grains improve the immune system, it also helps protect the cells from free radicals. Moreover, the soluble part of the fibers is beneficial for intestinal flora.

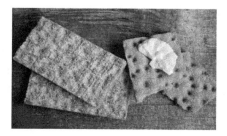

Contraindications

The fibers contained in whole grains must be taken in moderation by people suffering from diseases such as colitis and irritable bowel syndrome. In these situations, the intestinal mucus is more sensitive, and the dietary fibers risk aggravating the symptoms.

Chapter 2: What Is the Whole Food Diet?

With the progress of medical research, much time has been spent to identify the perfect diet to improve one's health and well-being. Studies have shown that the eating habits of our ancestors, some hundreds or even thousands of years ago, were more efficient in providing the nutrients that are suitable for the body. The idea of having a diet composed of whole foods came from this discovery. But what is the whole foods diet? In this chapter, we will spend some time talking about the main principles behind it.

What exactly is a whole foods nutritional regimen?

If we listen to nutrition experts, they will say that it is healthier to consume foods in their natural form or, in any case, as close to natural as possible. Modern eating habits and an unhealthy way of living has negatively affected our shape, especially if we consider the fact that, nowadays, there are a lot of overweight people. This has led the general public's interest in dieting to increase, and in particular, towards whole foods.

The following suggestions and ideas were written with the intent of helping you understand the diet of whole foods and to guide you on how you can apply it effectively.

The raw foods list is made up of unprocessed meat, raw cereals, fresh vegetables, fruit, unprocessed fish and non-homogenized milk. In general, a lot of credit and attention is given to fruits and vegetables, which have a lot of nutrients.

During the whole food diet, we strongly recommend to stay away from supplements and consume high quantities of fruits and veggies instead. As research has demonstrated many times, these foods can provide the body with all the nutrients it could possibly need.

Instead of eating processed grains, use whole grain products. In fact, processed grains, even if they taste better, are very low on fibers and don't offer high-quality nutrients.

Also, we kindly recommend you to not consume white flour and white sugar. If you cannot resist, just limit your consumption as much as possible. Research has shown that, when compared to whole wheat flour, white flour has a negligible amount of dietary fiber which is fundamental for maintaining an efficient digestive system.

We recommend you that you eat as many salads and mixed fruit bowls as you can. They are not only good for the entire body, but they taste fantastic as well. Variety is key, so keep experimenting to keep the taste fresh and new every time. During the whole food diet regimen, it is advisable to eat fruits for breakfast and avoid sweet treats. There is no need to buy expensive fruits all the time, especially when you get local fruits. If you live in an area where you can these fruits easily, try to get to know which vendor has the best products.

When it comes to beverages, consuming large quantities of soft drinks, beer, and cocktails is obviously not healthy. Instead, try to substitute them with clear water. You will notice the difference quite fast.

Smoothies are something that could really help you lose weight. We highly advise them, especially during the summer where you might not feel like eating solid food.

Any type of beans is better when it is not unrefined, so we suggest you avoid processed versions of them. In fact, when they are processed, they lose a lot of their nutritional values which is something you want to avoid.

You will be astonished to discover that the meals you can eat during the whole food diet are extremely simple to prepare and the ingredients are easy to find. If you have a lot of time you can dedicate to food preparation, it's better if you use your imagination and spend most of it trying to create new combinations or recipes.

Below are some simple meals that are very easy to prepare:

Potatoes with sour cream

This dish is perfect as a healthy snack. The process is extremely simple:

1. Just bake the potatoes (white or red).
2. Sprinkle them with the type of salt that you like the most.
3. Serve them with fresh and crispy onions.
4. If you want to add a little bit of extra taste, then try to serve them with a little sour cream on the side. You are going to love it.

Grilled chicken with baked potatoes

If you are looking for a tasty first meal, try this recipe. Here are the steps:

1. Grill a fair portion of chicken and use baked potatoes as a side dish.
2. Add flavored salt (in this case a flavored ingredient is allowed) and a little bit of mayonnaise for an amazing experience. Do not add too much because mayonnaise contains a lot of fat.

Whole pasta with pesto

1. Prepare a portion of whole pasta and add some organic pesto (better if it's homemade).
2. If you want, you can even slice up some tomatoes and add them at the end, to give yourself some vitamins as well.

There are a lot of dishes that you can try, just remember what is allowed and what is better to avoid.

Chapter 3: The Main Whole Grains

There are 11 kinds of whole grains, do you know them all?

For a balanced diet, it is advisable to eat the food allowed on this diet in rotation as they have different nutritional principles, we can find them in the form of grains, wholemeal flour, or brown beans.

In short, the main whole grains are rye, oats, millet, wheat, spelt, rice, barley, and kamut, most of them are gluten-free.

The other 3 (quinoa, buckwheat, and amaranth) are pseudo-cereals. They are not cereals, but they do have quality fibers and carbohydrates. Not to mention, they are, all gluten-free!

Let's discuss the whole grains one by one, what they contain, and how to cook them:

Millet

Millet contains essential minerals, such as iron, phosphorus, magnesium, zinc, selenium, and potassium. Naturally gluten-free, it can be consumed blown or in grains, and it contains more proteins than rice. This is a kind of totally natural supplement.

Whole grain rice

The whole rice differs from the white one as it preserves the outer layers of the grain that are 'scraped' away to obtain the usual rice.

It is richer because it has more fibers that help restore and keep intestinal flora in balance, it is also rich in minerals such as silicon, potassium phosphorus, magnesium, and B vitamins. Naturally, it's also gluten-free.

Grain or wheat

For most people, it is the best kind of cereal, and it's also the most present in the diet in the form of bread, pasta, and pizza.

It contains vitamins E, B6, B3, and beta-carotene, and protects us against free radicals.
It's used to make pasta or flour but is normally used to make sweet and savory baked goods. It contains gluten, however.

Quinoa

Quinoa is gluten-free, counteracts aging, helps fight cellular inflammation and is rich in calcium.

Kamut

Also known as Khorasan wheat, the kamut contains 20 to 40% more protein than wheat, contains more lipids, mineral salts (selenium, zinc, and magnesium), and vitamins. Kamut flour is used to make biscuits, bread, pasta, and cakes. It contains gluten.

Oats

Oats are the whole grains (potassium and 13% protein) which have the highest amount of nutrition. The fibers you can get from oats protect the layers of mucus found in the intestine and fights constipation. Oats are excellent with yogurt and milk, and it's a perfect breakfast or a healthy snack, even for athletes who follow a strict eating regimen. Oats can also be eaten with steamed or boiled vegetables.

Amaranth

Similar to millet in terms of nutritional intake, but it contains more fibers, iron, calcium, and lysine. Amaranth comes in the form of grains or even flour. It does not contain gluten.

Corn

Corn is gluten-free, which is why it can be eaten by people with celiac disease, but it is not a good source of vitamins. However, it contains vitamins B1, B6, iron, and magnesium.

Barley

Barley is a great source of lysine, vitamins B1, B2, PP, and calcium. The barley grain can be whole or refined. Excellent if consumed with vegetable soups. It contains gluten though.

Spelt

Rich in proteins, fibers, and vitamins compared to wheat, but it contains gluten. Spelt is suitable for diabetics and sportsmen because of its high magnesium content.

Rye

Similar to wheat, rich in fiber, but has less protein. And, it contains gluten. Its commonly used to make bread.

Chapter 4: The Whole 30 Challenge

Once you start the diet, you may feel doubt it because it's most likely that you've already tried meal plans in the past which didn't work. Time and time again, new fads and trends will come from the diet industry promising healthy and quick weight loss. After all, this is the secret dream of every person who goes on a diet instead of enjoying an excellent cup of ice cream.

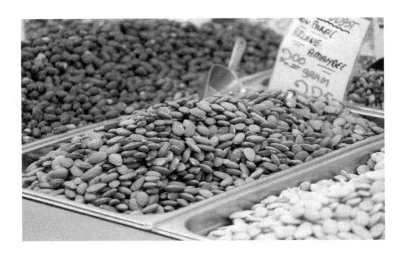

These days, the latest trend is called Whole 30, a diet based on the famous Paleo diet. The difference is that fruits and vegetables were added, promising a weight loss of up to 10 kg in 30 days. This is a food regime that was developed by two American nutritionists and is incredibly popular, especially among teenagers.

According to Melissa and Dallas Hartwig, the creators of the diet, if this way of eating is followed for at least 30 days, it will not only make the body slimmer, but it will also detoxify one's system. In this meal plan, any kind of food which only prove to be harmful or make you gain excessive weight is completely abolished.

But how does the Whole 30 work? First of all, there is no a weekly menu to follow. You only have a guide on what you should eat and how much should be eaten to completely avoid food that's banned from the diet. Included in the list of banned things are alcohol, smoking, sugar, and dairy products as well as cereals and legumes. This is something that's already seen in many other diet plans, but the Whole 30 diet plan has one major exception. In this diet plan, fruits and vegetables are not only accepted in moderate quantities but are greatly recommended as well.

The foods allowed are meat, fish, eggs, vegetables, and fruits, both fresh and dried. Unlike other diets, fruits and vegetables can be consumed. You can eat potatoes (as long as they are not fried), coconuts, olives, walnuts, pistachios, etc. And to make things even better, iodized salt, vinegar, and clarified butter are allowed. In addition, fish oil, vitamin D, probiotics, and magnesium are also recommended.

Now, let's have a look at how we can follow this diet. To make it work, according to the designers, it is necessary to follow this way of eating for 30 consecutive days without any exception. Forbidden foods must not be eaten for any reason. Using the food that's permitted on this diet, it's possible for you to create whatever recipe you want with them.

What to eat if you take the Whole 30 challenge

- **Breakfast**
  Scrambled eggs with a teaspoon of layered butter and almond milk without sugar

- **Snack**
  A handful of dried fruit

- **Lunch**
  Minestrone or grilled vegetables followed a small portion of grilled chicken

- **Snack**
  A fruit

- **Dinner**
  Roasted salmon with a side dish of potatoes

Pros and cons of this diet

Although it is not exactly a simple diet to follow, the Whole 30 has almost every food you can eat to gain proper nutrition. Unfortunately, these do not include cereals and legumes. Still, thirty days of following this diet will yield more results than taking another random diet plan or supplement. Ever more so, with the help of a nutritionist.

However, the stability of the diet is still in question. As to whether or not this restrictive diet can suppress the psychological effects of hunger while a person is losing weight has yet to be determined.

PART 4

Introduction

We are sick. As a society, America is very, very sick. If you have any doubts about how sick we are, look at how many medications are available to people without any prescription. How many medications are your friends and family taking? That number should be a wake-up call about the poor state of the health of Americans. If you are still in doubt, how many people do you know who struggle with cancer, heart disease, type 2 diabetes, depression, anxiety, infertility, or any other chronic diseases? One or two generations ago, those problems were virtually nonexistent. Now, they are becoming more the norm rather than the exception.

Medication is able to mask the symptoms of the diseases that we face. Statins can lower cholesterol but are unable to reverse heart disease or heal the body so that it is able to regulate its own cholesterol levels. Antidepressants can boost levels of serotonin, the "feel good" hormone, but are unable to heal the brain. In addition, medications come with a host of side effects that can cause other health problems, leading to a perceived need for more medication. The cause of these diseases is something that medication is unable to treat: poor diet. Aristotle, however, is credited with saying that food should be your medicine. The plant-based diet is a way to treat the cause of disease rather than medicating away the symptoms. It is just what America needs to regain its health.

Chapter 1: Obesity and the Standard American Diet

The Obesity Epidemic

There is no question that America is facing an obesity epidemic. An epidemic is a medical crisis that affects large parts of a population. With approximately eighty million adults and fifteen million children dealing with obesity, it has become one of the biggest health concerns today.

There is much more to obesity than being fat because obesity leads to many health problems. It is often correlated with high levels of blood sugar and insulin resistance, which, left unchecked, lead to type 2 diabetes. Excess fat in the abdominal area puts extra strain on the lumbar spine; in fact, just ten extra pounds of abdominal fat creates the equivalent of a hundred pounds of pressure on the spine. For this reason, obese people tend to suffer from back pain, sometimes to the extent that their daily routines and quality of life are affected. Extra fat places strain on the skeleton, leading many obese people to suffer from joint problems, particularly in the ankles, which bear most of the body's weight. The excess fat can build up in the blood vessels and visceral organs, leading to problems such as cardiovascular disease (including high blood pressure, heart attack, stroke, coronary artery disease, and congestive heart failure), respiratory difficulty, and fatty liver disease (which can mimic the effects of long-term alcohol abuse). Obesity can lead to hormonal disruptions, which can cause problems such as acne, polycystic ovary syndrome (PCOS) in women, and metabolic syndrome (a condition in which the body's ability to carry out its basic functions is compromised). Obese people are also more prone to sleep problems, such as sleep apnea, which occurs when the airway becomes partially blocked, causing the person to consistently wake up throughout the night. In addition to the physical problems, people who are obese also tend to struggle with emotional issues. These include challenges with self-esteem, body image, and social anxiety. Clearly, obesity is a problem that needs to be addressed and taken seriously.

While other components, such as genetics or metabolic disorders, may play a role in obesity, the main culprit leading to obesity is lifestyle choices, chiefly diet and exercise. In the nineteenth and early twentieth centuries, Americans were much more active because their lifestyles required it. People who worked on farms would be up milking cows, plowing fields, baling hay, planting crops, and harvesting from sunup to sundown. Think for a minute about how much physical energy farm work consumes! In the cities, most people did not have access to automated transportation, such as cars. Therefore, they mostly walked to their destinations, including work, school, and the grocery store. Furthermore, they did not have processed foods but only fruits, vegetables, grains, dairy, nuts, and meat that came from farms.

Today, many Americans have largely sedentary lifestyles. They drive to work, take the elevator instead of walking up the stairs, sit in chairs at their desks all day, drive home, and then watch television. Instead of bringing a healthy meal from home, many go out to eat for lunch, filling their diets with processed food and lots of sugar and little fiber (even if the food is labeled as healthy). With people getting little to no fiber, the sugar gets into the bloodstream, causing a sharp rise in insulin. High levels of insulin are linked to metabolic syndrome, weight gain, hormonal imbalances (insulin itself is a hormone), and diabetes. Instead of getting burned off through exercise, the sugar goes into the body's cells — usually much, much more than the cells require — and becomes converted into fat. Years of abusing the body through poor diet choices and lack of exercise lead to disease and a marked decrease in quality of life for individuals. As a society, it leads to a crippling burden on the medical system, causing resources (personnel, research dollars, lab equipment, etc.) that could be used to research and treat other conditions (such as pediatric cancer or spinal cord injuries) to be disproportionately allocated to treat the diseases associated with obesity.

Note that the text said "the diseases associated with obesity." The modern medical system is not as interested in treating obesity, the underlying cause of many of the diseases. The fact is that you cannot medicate yourself into health. A doctor cannot prescribe a pill that will make a patient healthy. The battle against obesity begins not in the doctor's office but in the kitchen, with the foods that people eat.

Why Are We so Fat?

The number one culprit behind the unprecedented weight gain of Americans is sugar. So many of the foods that we eat contain large amounts of added sugar; this is not only referring to sweets. Things as seemingly innocent as tomato soup and salad dressing are loaded with extra sugar. Americans consume far, far too much sugar.

The Problem with Calories

The problem with calories is essentially twofold. The first problem is that many people are not able to properly use the calories that they consume. Calories are necessary for the body to be able to function optimally. Calories are units of energy, so ideally, the number of calories that you consume will determine how much energy you have. However, the situation for many people is different, as their bodies lack the necessary vitamins and minerals needed to process that energy. That is why you may feel sluggish and tired after eating a large slice of cake (following the sugar rush, of course), which is high in calories but virtually devoid of nutrients.

The second problem with calories is that most Americans consume far, far too many of them. Not only are they not only able to properly use their calories, but the excessive number indirectly leads to weight gain. Notice that this said "indirectly" leads to weight gain, as calories themselves are not the culprit. Rather, the foods that contain the inordinate number of calories are to blame. Foods that are high in calories tend to be heavily processed and devoid of nutrients and come in supersized portions. For example, a hamburger found in a kid's happy meal is actually closer to how much an adult should consume; meanwhile, the kids eat the adult-sized hamburger while the adults eat the massive Big Mac and wash it down with a milkshake. Even processed foods that are low-calorie are deceptive, as they are also devoid of nutrients, largely unsatisfying (causing many people to consume far more than one serving), and can lead to weight gain. Nutritious foods, such as fresh fruits and vegetables, grass-fed beef, and free-range poultry are not only lower in calories than processed food but also much higher in nutrients, causing you to eat less. People who eat these foods feel full sooner, are more satisfied, and are all-around healthier.

The fact is that not all calories are created equal. One gram of sugar has four calories, while one gram of fat has nine calories. Simple arithmetic says to eat foods high in sugar rather than foods high in fat. However, this overly simplistic solution overlooks how our bodies actually use calories. Processed sugar is not necessary for the body to properly function; rather, it is hugely detrimental. In addition, if sugar is not immediately burned off, it quickly turns into fat. Furthermore, sugar has consistently been proven to actually increase someone's appetite, causing the person to consume far more than he or she normally would. While fat has more calories than sugar, there are some good types of fat that your body needs to be able to function properly. These include some saturated fats (found in free-range, grass-fed, organic animal products such as milk, beef, and eggs), omega-3 fatty acids (found in eggs and nuts), and monounsaturated fat (found in nuts and avocados). The body responds to these fats in vastly different ways than it responds to the lab-created fats — such as hydrogenated oils — found in processed foods. Eating good fats causes you to feel full, leading you to actually consume fewer calories while giving your body what it needs.

All of this is to say that instead of counting calories, what you really should be doing is paying more attention to the foods that contain those calories.

The American Diet

The typical American diet relies too much on convenience, so much so that people are willing to compromise their own physical health rather than be bothered with worrying about what they are eating. Breakfast food options in many supermarkets are centered on convenience rather than nutrition: sugary cereals, Pop-tarts, frozen breakfast sandwiches, and instant oatmeal. Most of these processed options have had most of their nutritional contents removed (instant oatmeal has far less fiber and other nutrients than steel-cut oats) and lots of sugar added. They are also devoid of fresh fruit (despite many of the claims on packages). Sadly, many people consume these products rather than making a nutritious breakfast that includes fresh fruit and protein. When office workers go out to lunch every day rather than bringing a healthy, pre-packed lunch from home, the reason is usually because going to a restaurant is more convenient than waking up fifteen minutes earlier. Going to a drive-through after a long day of work is so much more convenient than preparing a nutritious meal from scratch.

The result of all this convenience is way, way too many carbs, too much sodium, and too much unhealthy fat, such as hydrogenated oils, and far too few nutrients, such as vitamins, minerals, and fiber. Some people think that they can correct this imbalance by taking a multivitamin and fiber supplement every morning. However, the quality of the vitamins and minerals in supplements is of lower quality than of those found in fresh food, and they don't exist in the natural combination that our bodies require for optimal processing. In fact, the body only absorbs about ten to twenty percent of the nutrients found in a multivitamin. Fiber supplements can be of assistance, especially to people who are elderly but cannot produce all the benefits of including fiber in the diet throughout the day. Those benefits include lower levels of blood sugar and insulin and feeling full for longer.

What may be shocking to many people is that a lot of Americans are malnourished! This type of malnourishment is not the result of an inadequate amount of food but by poor food choices. Furthermore, excessive sugar actually reduces the body's ability to absorb the nutrients that it does receive. Many Americans have critically low levels of crucial vitamins such as D, K, and the B complex, which prohibit their bodies from being able to function optimally. This is yet another reason why so many people are sick.

Abdominal Fat Problem: Fastest Place to Lose Weight

One of the most dangerous places for the body to store fat is in the abdominal area; excess abdominal fat is so dangerous that it is actually a predictor of conditions such as heart disease and type 2 diabetes. The good news is that abdominal fat is the easiest type to lose. You don't have to do crunches or sit-ups to lose it; rather, you simply need to change your diet.

Abdominal fat is created by poor diet choices, such as excessive sugar, alcohol, and processed foods that contain unhealthy fats. In order to start losing it, eat foods that are low in sugar and other refined carbs, high in fiber, and high in protein. Examples include fresh fruits and vegetables, homemade soups and stews, and nuts and seeds. To further fight the belly bulge, rather than doing abdominal exercises, the best exercise to do is cardio, such as brisk walking and swimming.

Problems and Trappings of a High-Carb Diet

Americans consume far, far too much sugar and other refined carbs. Even though carbs are lower in calories than fats, they lead to weight gain. Refined carbs actually "flip a switch" inside the brain that signals that you need to keep eating more carbs. Furthermore, a few hours afterward, you may have a craving to eat more carbs. As a result, you end up consuming an excessive amount of empty calories instead of giving your body the nutrition that it needs.

In summary, Americans are facing an unprecedented health crisis brought on not by lack of food, but by an overabundance of food. Americans are consuming far too many calories, but are actually malnourished because the calories that they consume are not filled with the nutrients that they need for their bodies to function properly. Furthermore, too many Americans lack an understanding of what calories really are and what our bodies need in order to use them as energy. As a result, much of the population is fat and sick.

Chapter 2: Knowledge about Proper Nutrition

What Causes High Blood Sugar and High Blood Pressure?

High blood sugar exists when the bloodstream is filled with more sugar than it can process. When sugar enters the bloodstream, insulin is secreted by the pancreas to enable the body's cells to absorb the sugar and use it for energy. However, if there is more sugar in the bloodstream than the cells need, it builds up and insulin levels remain high. Over time, high insulin levels cause the cells to stop responding to it as efficiently, so more is required for them to absorb the sugar from the blood. If this is not corrected, the result can be insulin resistance. Insulin resistance will cause blood sugar levels to remain high, no matter how much insulin is secreted. If left untreated, diabetes can ensue.

The cause of high blood sugar is simple: too much sugar and not enough fiber in the diet. When sugar is consumed with fiber — for example, in fresh fruit, which contains sugar but also contains fiber — it released into the bloodstream more slowly, giving the body time to allow the cells to absorb it. However, when sugar is consumed without any fiber — for example, in a soda or piece of cake — it jets into the bloodstream, causing blood sugar levels to rise.

Blood pressure refers to the force of blood pressing against the walls of blood vessels; high blood pressure means that the blood is pressing too hard, which, over time, can cause damage to the cardiovascular system. The blood vessels can become stiff and hard, a sometimes fatal condition referred to as atherosclerosis. Poor diet choices are also behind many cases of high blood pressure. While there is a genetic component for *some* cases of high blood pressure, it is more often than not linked to the typical American diet. Rather than being linked to excessive sugar intake, high blood pressure seems to be more associated with excessive salt (most processed foods have very high levels of sodium) and bad fats, such as hydrogenated oils.

Lectins and Why They Are Bad

Lectins are proteins that bind to both cell membranes and sugar. They are found in nearly all plants and animals because they help cells communicate with each other. However, they can be very dangerous. One reason why is that some lectins are extremely toxic. For example, ricin, a toxin that is fatal in extremely small amounts, is derived from the lectins found in the castor bean.

Another reason why lectins are so dangerous is that they cause inflammation. Inflammation is one of the body's natural defenses against infection and other foreign invaders. However, over time, inflammation can lead to heart disease, hormonal disruptions, aches and pains, and a host of other problems. In addition, lectins can contribute to leaky gut syndrome, something that will be explained in detail in Chapter 7.

Lectins are found in nearly all of the foods that we consume. However, the biggest culprits include white potatoes, eggplant, beans, and dairy. Dairy poses a double danger because it is actually designed to penetrate the lining of the intestine, the cause of the leaky gut syndrome. These seemingly healthy foods should be avoided at all costs.

In summary, many Americans struggle with high blood sugar and high blood pressure. However, they do not understand how their poor diets and lifestyle choices are actually creating these problems. High blood sugar and high blood pressure are caused by consuming sugary processed food; high blood pressure is also the result of eating too much meat. These conditions can actually be reversed by changing eating patterns. In addition, lectins are proteins found in nearly all foods but are toxic, especially when consumed in large amounts. While plant-based foods should be consumed in favor of processed foods and meat, special care should be taken to avoid lectins.

Chapter 3: Lack of Exercise

Have you ever bought a gym membership at the beginning of the year? Gyms tend to heavily discount their memberships to entice the hordes of people making New Year's resolutions about getting fit and losing weight. They aren't taking a risk by offering their product/service at a rate that is too low because they know that within a month, most of the people who bought a membership will forget that they even have it. Most of those gym memberships will be used for a few weeks before being forgotten for the rest of the year.

This highlights the fact that Americans get far too little exercise. Our lifestyles have become quite sedentary, exemplified by the long hours that we sit at desks using computers (both at work and at home) and how much time we spend watching television. While for our ancestors' exercise was built into their daily routines, through activities such as hunting, farming, and walking long distances, we don't really need to exercise to get through the day. There are exceptions, such as occupations that require people to be on their feet constantly or those that involve heavy labor. However, for the most part, we are able to get through our lives just fine without any exercise. This lack of exercise is taking a huge toll on the nation's health. Not only are we consuming far too much sugar and processed foods, but we are not burning off any of those excessive calories.

The benefits of exercise beyond burning calories are tremendous. Exercise releases endorphins, which boost the mood; therefore, exercise is nature's own antidepressant. Chronic stress, something that many Americans struggle with (some without even realizing it, because stress has become such a normal part of life), causes hormones such as cortisol and adrenaline to be released into the bloodstream. High levels of cortisol are known to lead to weight gain, especially in the abdominal area. Exercise, however, burns off cortisol and other hormones that, over time, can cause damage. Exercise helps people sleep better at night, improves heart health, regulates and even decreases appetite, produces more mental clarity, lowers blood pressure, and burns off excessive blood sugar. With all of these benefits, in addition to burning calories, it is a wonder that exercise is not prescribed more than medication!

In summary, the benefits of exercise cannot be overstated. It increases bone and muscle strength, strengthens the heart, improves blood flow, and boosts mood. However, too many Americans lead largely sedentary lives that are practically devoid of exercise. As a result, their bodies are not able to function properly and they are chronically lethargic and fatigued. Instead of dealing with the root of the problem — lack of exercise — many opt for expensive and dangerous medications.

Chapter 4: Downfall of Medication

When is the last time you saw a commercial or online advertisement about lawsuits for people who took a certain medication and experienced dangerous side effects? When is the last time you saw a commercial or online advertisement for a particular medication, and in the fine print was a list of dozens of harmful side effects, some of which could be life-threatening? Up until 1985, advertising prescription medications directly to consumers rather than to doctors was illegal. However, nowadays our media is inundated with ads for prescription medications, and as a society, we have become fixated on the idea that a pill can cure most, if not all, of our ailments.

What Medication Does to Your Body

The reality is that while medication can alleviate some symptoms and be very beneficial in critical cases, it can also be very damaging to the body. This section will look at different types of medication and the harm that they can cause.

Antidepressants. Approximately 10% of the US population is on antidepressants, and they are the third most prescribed category of medication. Most antidepressants work by preventing neurons from reabsorbing the hormone serotonin, the "feel-good" hormone. This raises overall serotonin levels, but over time, causes an imbalance of serotonin inside and outside of neurons. Because serotonin does more than elevating mood (it also aids in the growth and death of neurons, digestion, reproduction, and blood clotting), imbalanced levels can lead to problems such as digestive problems (including abdominal bleeding), sexual dysfunction, and sleep disturbances. Furthermore, after prolonged use (even just a few months), the brain begins to push back after the effects of the drug in order to restore the proper balance of serotonin. This can lead to a full-blown relapse of depression, even while people are still taking the medication. Commonly, doctors will either increase the dose or switch patients to a stronger antidepressant without appreciating that the brain itself is working against the drug.

Painkillers. Painkillers are usually taken in the form of over-the-counter medication to alleviate discomfort associated with aches and pains, including menstrual cramps and arthritis. While many people are aware of the dangers of narcotic painkillers, even OTC ones are harmful. They work by preventing nerves from being able to carry out their functions, namely, to transmit messages from different parts of the body to the brain. Long-term use can actually lead to nerve damage. In addition, they are harmful to the liver and can cause stomach bleeding, which can be fatal.

Antibiotics. Antibiotics are commonly prescribed to treat bacterial infections, such as respiratory infections. They work by killing off the bacteria inside the body. However, the body naturally contains good bacteria, including approximately five pounds of it in the gut alone! This gut bacteria are known as the microbiome and are essential to carrying out many vital functions, including absorption of nutrients and regulation of hormones. Because antibiotics are indiscriminate in the bacteria that they kill, they devastate the microbiome and therefore disrupt many of the body's natural processes.

In addition, strains of bacteria are becoming resistant to antibiotics. This is because as a nation, we have become so dependent on medications, believing that a pill can fix all of our health problems, that we have overused antibiotics. Some patients are so insistent on getting medicated for whatever ailments they have that they are prescribed antibiotics for viruses, such as colds, something that antibiotics are powerless against. In response, the bacteria develop defenses to protect them from the antibiotics. The result is that new and difficult-to-treat diseases, such as MRSA, are becoming increasingly common.

Ultimately, medication is able to alleviate the symptoms of the disease, but it is not able to cure the overall dysfunction that led to the problem. Statins can lower cholesterol, but they cannot fix the cause of high cholesterol: poor diet and lack of exercise. Antibiotics can fight off foreign invaders that lead to infection, but they cannot heal the body so that it is able to defend itself through its natural mechanisms without antibiotics. If you want to actually address the cause of your symptoms rather than become a revolving-door patient, you need to fix and change your diet.

In summary, there is no benefit that medication can provide that adequate nutrition and exercise cannot provide, but without the damaging side effects. Exercise is more effective at treating depression and anxiety than antidepressants and other mood-enhancing medications. Having an optimized microbiome in the gut, fed with plenty of high-fiber fruits, vegetables, and probiotics, cannot only treat infections better than antibiotics but can eliminate the pathogens before they even take hold. Our lifestyles are what have made us sick, and medication cannot fix a lifestyle problem. Medications are dangerous and produce side effects that can pose long-term health risks. A healthy plant-based diet, however, can replace the need for medication

Chapter 5: Case Studies of Places with the Highest Longevity

Despite its reputation for being wealthy and prosperous, the United States actually ranks number 50 in the world in terms of life expectancy, with Americans living an average of just over 78 years. Countries that fare better have several things in common, including social factors that cause people to lead healthier lifestyles. The world's highest life expectancy — nearly 90 years — is found in Monaco, which also has the world's highest population of millionaires and billionaires. Since most of the rest of us can't afford the kind of lifestyle that may contribute to the high longevity of residents of Monaco, that and other small, wealthy states will be disregarded.

Okinawa, Japan. The Japanese inhabitants of the island of Okinawa eat a low-fat diet that largely consists of fish, tofu, seaweed, and vegetables. Many of them actually only consume 1200 calories a day; however, their life expectancy is approximately 87 years, three years longer than their other Japanese compatriots. In fact, Okinawa has five times as many centenarians as the rest of Japan! Many Okinawans remain healthy until the end of their lives, and those who are 80 years old may have bodies that more closely resemble that of someone in his or her forties or fifties.

Loma Linda, California. Loma Linda is a small town of about 25,000 people, about sixty miles from Los Angeles. It is the center of the Seventh-Day Adventist Church, which advocates a plant-based diet and strongly discourages smoking. The different lifestyle habits of the church's members may be what contributes to the fact that its residents enjoy a life expectancy of about 85 years, as compared to the rest of the United States, which is only about 78 years.

Iceland. The small Nordic country of Iceland has an average life expectancy of just under 83 years, the highest in Europe. It also has exceptionally low infant mortality. These results can be at least partially attributed to the clean energy used to provide for the nation's power needs. However, they can also be attributed to the traditional diet of Iceland, which is high in fish, and a culture that promotes being physically active, especially outdoors.

In summary, cultures that promote the highest rates of longevity have several things in common. The people tend to be more active than in other parts of the world, thereby reaping the myriad benefits of exercise. Their diets are low in meat and other animal products and high in fruits and vegetables.

Chapter 6: Who This Book Is For

If you are struggling with any health problems, even those that may be genetic, then this book is for you. This chapter will look at what the plant-based diet can do for many common health problems.

Autoimmune disease. An autoimmune disease results when the body's immune system believes that healthy cells are foreign invaders and attacks them as such. Examples of autoimmune diseases include Crohn's, rheumatoid arthritis, and multiple sclerosis. Chronic inflammation is believed to be one of the causes; in fact, it is the culprit behind many chronic diseases. Inflammation is triggered by foods high in sugar and excessive consumption of meat, especially processed meat. Eating a diet mostly from plants results not only in less inflammation but a reversal of the damage caused by long-term inflammation! Many people with autoimmune diseases who have switched to a plant-based diet have noticed not only that their symptoms are largely alleviated but also that the disease itself becomes reversed.

Irritable bowel syndrome (IBS). IBS is a condition that affects as much as 15% of the American population; it results in intestinal dysfunction, including cramping, bloating, diarrhea, abdominal pain, gas, and constipation. Eating a plant-based diet has proven to considerably help people with IBS. Fresh fruits and vegetables are high in prebiotics, which promote a healthy environment for the good bacteria that make up the colon's microbiome. Proper functioning of the microbiome is essential to bowel health, as well as the health of the rest of the body.

Brain fog. Brain fog, or a generalized lack of clarity, can be substantially helped by eating a plant-based diet. When your body is out of whack, usually caused by poor diet choices and lack of exercise, your mood and thinking can be dramatically affected. Giving your body the nutrition that it needs will ameliorate most, if not all of the problems that are contributing to fuzzy and clouded thinking as well as a depressed mood.

Arthritis. Arthritis, a painful joint condition, is caused largely by chronic inflammation in the joints. As previously stated, inflammation is caused by eating a diet high in refined carbs, especially sugars, and meat, especially processed meat. However, a plant-based diet will not only bring down inflammation but can actually reduce the damage caused by long-term chronic inflammation.

High blood pressure. Eating a lot of salt, as part of a diet high in processed food and low in fruits and vegetables, is the primary contributing factor to high blood pressure. Studies have shown that reduced consumption of meat — consuming only one or two servings a week — resulted in most participants, blood pressure was reduced by about 25%. This result was achieved without a drug supplement. Going to a full vegetarian diet reduced blood pressure by up to 40%.

High cholesterol. Cholesterol is found exclusively in animal products. Plants on their own do not produce cholesterol. Our bodies naturally produce some cholesterol, which is generally considered to be of the beneficial type. However, high consumption of meat and products derived from animals, results in high levels of bad cholesterol, which can lead to heart disease and other problems. Switching to a plant-based diet will naturally lower your cholesterol levels simply because you won't be consuming nearly as much.

Heart disease. The reason that heart disease is the primary cause of death in America is because of poor diets and lack of exercise. Americans fill their days with sedentary activities and lots of processed, sugary foods that are also high in sodium. Eating much less meat, especially red meat, eliminating sugar and processed food, and eating mostly vegetable- and fruit-based foods have been shown to dramatically lower rates of heart disease and even reverse it in people who already suffer from it.

Acid reflux. Acid reflux is a condition in which stomach acid is propelled upwards into the esophagus, causing a burning sensation. While one out of five Americans suffers from acid reflux, in rural African villages, the risk was only one in one thousand, making it virtually unheard of. Most foods in the American diet are highly acidic, thereby contributing to the symptoms. However, plant-based foods are more alkaline, or basic, and bases neutralize acids.

Overweight or obese. People who are overweight or obese and switch to a plant-based diet, rather than relying on low-calorie processed foods, lose much more weight. Feeding your body what it needs, instead of what tastes better, results in feelings of fullness, satiation, and fewer calories consumed. Further, because those calories are useful and used efficiently by the body, people have more energy and are able to exercise more.

Those who want to look healthier. When people want to brighten their complexions, look younger, and generally look healthier, they usually go to a salon for an expensive treatment or buy a skin cream. While these procedures may make people look healthier, true health comes from the inside and is reflected in the outer appearance. In other words, when people are healthy on the inside, they look healthy on the outside.

Reverse aging. Processed foods loaded with chemicals and sugar, along with large amounts of meat and dairy, cause our bodies to age faster. However, a plant-based diet can actually reverse some of the signs and symptoms of aging. While it can't reverse the aging process, it can slow it down. Telomeres are structures at the end of our cells' DNA that keep the double-helix structure from unwinding. Every time a cell divides, the telomere is weakened, leading to the effects of aging. Telomerase is an enzyme that helps rebuild telomeres, and a plant-based diet is linked with stronger telomerase activity. What this means is that a plant-based diet can help reverse some of the effects of aging and even slow the aging process.

In summary, many of the diseases that plague modern society are the direct result of poor lifestyle choices. Changing the way that we eat can reverse and even eliminate not only short-term infections and other acute diseases but also chronic diseases, as well. All of this is to say that whoever you are, whatever health problems you may be struggling with, the plant-based miracle diet is for you.

Chapter 7: Leaky Gut Syndrome

What is Leaky Gut Syndrome?

Leaky gut syndrome, like obesity, is becoming a national epidemic due to poor foot choices by much of the American population. The leaky gut syndrome has also been called intestinal hyperpermeability. The walls of the intestine are porous so that the nutrients in food can be absorbed into the bloodstream. However, in leaky gut, they become excessively porous, to the point that larger portions of undigested food, including waste and toxins, to enter the bloodstream. In response, the body begins to attack the foreign invaders. The liver works hard to filter out all of the food macromolecules but is unable to keep up with their constant flow into the bloodstream. The immune system then kicks in and attacks the macromolecules. They are then absorbed into the body's tissues, resulting in inflammation. As you have already seen, chronic inflammation is at the root of many diseases. Instead of carrying out its normal functions, such as filtering the blood and reducing inflammation, your body will actually go to war against itself, which can result in autoimmune disease.

Fungus Theory

Candida is a fungus that can live in your intestines; one theory about the origin of leaky gut syndrome is that it is the result of an overgrowth of candida. The theory states when a candida yeast infection grows unchecked, the fungus grows "roots" into the walls of the intestines. The wall of the intestine becomes overly porous, allowing large particles of undigested food to pass into the bloodstream.

Plant Protein

Protein from some plant sources, such as soy and wheat (wheat protein is gluten), should be avoided at all costs, as they are considered to be "anti-nutrients." Celiac disease, or gluten intolerance, is related to the leaky gut syndrome in that consuming gluten can actually lead to a 70% increase in intestinal permeability. Soy protein is just as bad; not only is 90% of soy genetically modified (which leads to a host of other problems) but on a molecular level, it mimics gluten. As a result, soy protein can also dramatically increase intestinal permeability.

Intestinal Irritants

Intestinal irritants can be behind many cases of leaky gut syndrome. There is no universal list of intestinal irritants; rather, the foods that should be avoided are, to some extent, particular to the individual. However, some of the most common culprits are caffeine, wheat (specifically, the gluten found in wheat), sugar, and soy. When foods that are intestinal irritants to you enter the bowel, they can pass through the bowel membrane and into the bloodstream.

To find what foods are problematic for you, eliminate consumption of one item at a time, for two weeks, and then gradually reintroduce it back into your diet to see what effect it has. For example, eliminate all dairy products for two weeks. Keep a journal to gauge whether you feel better or worse. At the end of two weeks, gradually begin consuming dairy again. Do you feel better or worse? If you feel worse when consuming it, dairy is probably an intestinal irritant for you.

There may be other foods that are intestinal irritants for you that are not on the general list. If you are still having problems, you may need to see a specialist to determine exactly what foods should be avoided, at least until your gut heals.

Lectin Plant Proteins

Lectins are proteins found in nearly all foods; they are produced by plants and therefore consumed by animals that eat plants. Thus, they make their way into the entire food system. Consumption of lectins cannot be avoided; however, you should try to limit them as much as possible, especially if you are dealing with leaky gut syndrome.

Lectins are problematic for leaky gut syndrome because they gravitate towards areas like the lining of the gut, where they attach themselves and cause intestinal damage. Eliminating all grains and soy, which tend to be very high in lectins, will help heal your gut. Once the lining is restored, you can gradually add back in grains that have been fermented and sprouted; these grains have smaller amounts of lectins.

Whole Grains and Resistant Starches

Whole grains are usually described as healthy. However, that is only partially true, as they may be healthier than their refined (white) counterparts in areas such as glycemic index. In fact, whole grain bread is higher in lectins than white bread because the refining process significantly reduces the amount of lectins. Consider that the grains harvested to make bread and other foods are actually the seeds of plants. If all of a plant's seeds were eaten, that plant would become extinct; therefore, nature evolved a way to prevent seeds from being eaten. Seeds have a hard shell that is lined with lectins and other anti-nutrients, to keep them from being eaten. This reason is why whole grains, even more than white grains, contribute to leaky gut syndrome.

Instead of whole grains, opt for sprouted grains. Sprouted grains have been allowed to germinate before being milled into flour, thereby eliminating the toxins contained in the shell of the seed. Sprouted grains have significantly fewer lectins but still retain the nutrient content (unlike white, refined grains). Many kinds of bread now, such as Ezekiel bread, are being made from sprouted grains.

Potatoes and beans are often heralded as "resistant starches," meaning that the starch isn't digested and the calories are not absorbed. However, potatoes, beans, and other resistant starches are high in saponin, which actually creates holes in the cells that line the intestines. Even just a small amount of the cellular damage created by saponins can prevent nutrients from being transported by the cells. Furthermore, these resistant starches contain something called protease inhibitors, which increase levels of trypsin. Trypsin is an enzyme that damages the connections between the cells that line the intestines, thereby increasing the gut's permeability.

In summary, leaky gut syndrome is one of the diseases plaguing modern society because it is caused by poor diet. It is behind many cases of inflammation, abdominal discomfort, autoimmune disease, and toxins in the blood. Leaky gut syndrome is brought on by eating foods high in lectins, including seemingly healthy whole grains and beans. It is also caused by eating genetically modified food, dairy, caffeine, and any other foods that may be particularly irritating to you as an individual.

All of this may sound like a long list of foods to be avoided. However, the plant-based miracle diet is more about increasing your palate and enjoying foods that you would never have even considered.

Chapter 8: The Plant-Based Miracle Diet

What is the Plant-Based Miracle Diet?

Rather than being an eating plan that you stick to for a set period of time, the plant-based miracle diet is essentially a revolution of lifestyle in which permanent lifestyle changes are made. Instead of opting for eating a certain number of calories each day or getting into an exercise regimen until certain results are achieved, the plant-based miracle diet is about eliminating all processed foods eating only whole foods or those that are minimally processed.

There are three forms of the plant-based miracle diet; whichever one you decide will depend on your body type, goals, and the lifestyle changes that you are willing to make. The first form allows for some consumption of meat, as long as it is only free-range, grass-fed, and organic. Modern farming methods aim to raise animals as quickly as possible so as to create the most profit for the food company; therefore, animals raised for their meat are fed subpar food that includes unused body parts from other animals, plastic pellets, and even manure. The animals often live in unhealthy conditions, being crammed into cages that are too small and living on top of each other. They aren't able to get any exercise, and as a result of these conditions, the animals themselves are sick. To keep them from getting sick and to help them grow faster, many animals are fed a steady stream of antibiotics (most antibiotics used today are for farming). Consider that anytime you eat conventional meat, you are consuming a sick animal. That reason alone is enough to make the switch to eating only meat that is organic, grass-fed, and free range. However, the bulk of the diet consists of fruits and vegetables, and meat is eaten no more than two or three times a week.

The second form of this diet is vegetarianism, which includes the consumption of wild-caught fish (rather than farmed fish, which are subject to many of the farming methods listed above) and organic eggs from free-range chickens or other poultry. The third form of this diet is complete veganism, in which absolutely no animal products are consumed.

Choosing what works for you may be a process in which you make some lifestyle changes, such as eating more fruits and vegetables while reducing your consumption of meat until you switch to vegetarianism. You may be entirely unable or unwilling to make the switch to vegetarianism, but you make sure that all of your meat is from healthy animals rather than those raised in a factory farm. You may already be a vegetarian but want to incorporate more fruits and vegetables into your diet until you transition all the way to veganism. Whichever choice is best for you, make sure that the changes you make are ones that you can and will stick with.

In addition to a significantly reduced meat consumption, the plant-based miracle diet is, well, about eating more plant-based foods. Conventional wisdom, such as the food pyramid, says that we should aim to eat five servings of fruits and vegetables a day. This mindset sets us up for the belief that we should add fruits and vegetables into the diet that we already consume, thereby making it healthy. For example, when eating out you may decide to substitute a side salad for fries, thereby making your meal healthy. However, nothing could be further from the truth. The side salad might add one serving of vegetables to a meal loaded with hydrogenated oil, refined carbohydrates, sugar, and trans fat. It can hardly begin to offset the damaging effects of this meal.

The entire diet actually needs to be overhauled, not to make room for more fruits and vegetables, but to make plant-based foods the foundation on which the entire diet is built. Instead of ordering a side salad with a hamburger or slice of pizza, the salad should be the main dish of the meal, possibly with a small amount of meat added as a topping. Instead of eating a bowl of cereal that claims to have fruit added, the fruit should be the centerpiece of breakfast. A bowl of fruit with sprouted-grain toast and an egg would be a much healthier, plant-based option.

Because so much of the American diet is built around convenience, making the change to a plant-based diet is not just changing the foods you eat but changing your entire lifestyle. You have to change the way that you think about food. Food is not meant to be convenient or something that you eat mindlessly throughout the day. Rather, it is the source from which your body derives its health. Aristotle is credited with saying that food should be your medicine. That should be your attitude about food.

If you must have coffee in the morning, instead of stopping by Starbucks on the way to work or even filling up at the office coffee pot, make a pot of organic coffee at home (coffee has some of the highest levels of pesticides and other chemicals of any crop in the world). Instead of going out to lunch because it is easier than preparing a lunch at home, make the lifestyle changes necessary in order to either prepare your lunch the night before or wake up ten minutes earlier so that you can prepare it in the morning. Invest in a slow cooker so that healthy soups and stews can cook while you are at work, and a healthy plant-based supper will be waiting for you when you get home.

The way that you shop for groceries will have to change. If you are used to clipping coupons and buying foods that are on sale, you will have to completely change how you think about buying food. Some foods, such as conventional, factory-farm milk and wheat-based products, are subsidized by the US government to keep the prices low for consumers while still giving the farmers a profit. However, as you have seen, these foods contribute to many of the health problems that are plaguing Americans today. Instead of opting for foods that are cheap or convenient, such as microwavable frozen dinners, go first to the organic part of the produce section. By far, the bulk of what you buy should be in this section.

Other options for procuring plant-based foods include going local. Farmers markets are great places to find produce and grass-fed meat that is raised by small, local farmers. While conventional produce may be grown on the other side of the world and picked before it is ripe so that it can be shipped to the United States, the produce at a farmer's market is usually picked either that day or the day before. Because small farmers are not usually subsidized and their costs tend to be higher than those of conventional farmers, the foods found at farmer's markets can be more expensive. If you qualify for programs such as WIC, they can help offset the cost. The quality of the food and value to the local economy, rather than big agricultural corporations, make the higher cost worth it.

Besides a farmer's market, you can also see if there are any pick-your-own farms in your area. A pick-your-own farm grows the produce, but local people go in and pick it. You pay after you are finished picking; the cost is based on the weight of produce that you picked. The farmers don't weigh you before and after, so you are free to eat as much as you want while you are out picking! Going to a pick-your-own farm can be a great family outing in which children learn more about food and where it comes from while being able to procure it for themselves. It will certainly be a different type of outing than a trip to the movies or a favorite restaurant!

As you can probably see, the plant-based diet involves more than simply changing what you eat. It is changing how you think about food and, in turn, making lifestyle changes to accommodate the new mindset.

Why Should You Get on This Diet?

As previously explained, many, if not most, of the health problems facing Americans today are related directly to the foods that they eat. Refined carbohydrates, especially sugar, cause a slew of problems ranging from metabolic syndrome, weight gain, and obesity, destruction of the microbiome, to insulin resistance and diabetes. Some have been tricked into believing that they can make a healthy switch from refined carbs to whole grains, such as swapping out their white bread for whole wheat bread. However, while whole grains have a lower glycemic index than refined carbs, they are high in lectins, which can damage the wall of the intestines and lead to leaky gut syndrome. Lack of adequate vitamins and minerals due to not eating enough fruits and vegetables causes problems with immunity, blood clotting, and other disorders that are commonly associated with malnutrition.

So many of these problems can be fixed — and are getting fixed — by getting onto the plant-based diet. Eliminating all processed foods and eating only whole foods is proving across the board to have a marked effect on people's health and even curing diseases, such as diabetes and terminal cancer, that were believed to be irreversible. Furthermore, a plant-based diet leads to higher levels of energy and a better mood, leading to an overall higher quality of life.

How to Attain a Clean Diet

Most of the foods that are grown through conventional methods are "dirty." This means that not only are the methods used to grow them very destructive to the environment (large amounts of wasted water, water being contaminated by sewage, large amounts of energy needed to transport them), but they are also loaded with pesticides and other chemicals that are not safe for human consumption. Many of the pesticides that the FDA has labeled "safe" are far more dangerous to both humans and the environment than the DDT that was outlawed in 1972.

In addition to high levels of pesticides, some major biotechnical companies, such as Monsanto and Syngenta, have manufactured genetically modified seeds. GMOs are touted as having unique benefits because of the DNA that was changed, allowing them to have properties such as being resistant to drought, having higher levels of certain vitamins, or being able to withstand the stronger pesticides sprayed on them. GMOs are so ubiquitous today that unless the label on your food says that it is organic or non-GMO, you can be certain that it does contain GMOs. GMOs are very harmful to human health on two main fronts. The first is that they contain particularly high levels of the dangerous pesticide glyphosate, which is a known carcinogen. The second is that it actually changes the DNA of some human cells and the bacteria that make up the gut's microbiome. It should come as no surprise that the rise of GMOs and the rise of the leaky gut syndrome have happened simultaneously. Furthermore, GMOs are incredibly destructive to the environment and have the potential to permanently alter the DNA of some species.

Many of these chemicals are stored in the liver, which acts as a filter. However, when the liver becomes overloaded because so many chemicals are entering our bodies, the chemicals are stored in fat cells. Because the body needs a place to store these toxins, it will refuse to get rid of excess fat cells. Losing weight can have as much to do with the chemicals in our food as with the food itself.

With this in mind, eating a plant-based diet is not enough. You need to ensure that the "healthy" whole foods that you are consuming are also clean, meaning free from these dangerous chemicals. The two ways to ensure that your food is not loaded with chemicals is to either make sure that it is labeled as GMO-free or organic or buy it locally from small farmers.

Scientific Mechanisms Behind the Plant-Based Diet

Genes are behind some of the diseases that we face. For example, some scientists have proposed that there is actually a genetic tendency for some people to gain weight easier and have a harder time losing it than other people. Some people are genetically more prone to addictive behaviors, such as smoking and overeating. Diseases such as cancer and Alzheimer's even have a genetic component! Genes are seen as an insurmountable obstacle to overcoming disease and attaining health and wellness. However, more and more studies are showing that a healthy lifestyle built around the plant-based diet can actually have more of an impact on disease, health, and well-being than genes.

In most cases, genes on their own do not cause disease (exceptions include childhood diseases such as cystic fibrosis). Rather, they predispose people to become more likely to develop a disease. For example, Mary Grace may have a gene that makes her more susceptible to developing breast cancer. All people have some number of cancerous cells in their bodies at all times, but they are usually destroyed by healthy cells that are properly functioning. Mary Grace's faulty gene may work in such a way that breast cells are more prone to turning into dangerous cancer cells, and the healthy remaining cells are less able to destroy the cancerous cells. That tendency can be either mitigated or augmented by her lifestyle. If she eats lots of damaging sugar and processed foods, her healthy cells will be even less capable of protecting her from cancerous cells. However, if she eats a diet that is based on organic, plant-based foods, she will be providing her healthy cells with the ability to fight off and destroy the cancerous cells. Furthermore, she will be giving the healthy cells the nutrients that they need to keep from mutating into cancerous cells in the first place. This example is just one way of how the plant-based miracle diet can override a person's genes and promote overall wellness.

In summary, the plant-based diet is a complete change of lifestyle, from one that is based on convenience and leads to disease, to one based on an understanding of health, well-being, and how certain foods contribute to an enhanced quality of life. It is not a list of foods that you can and can't eat, a point system, or measure of calories. You can't go to the grocery store and just buy a different brand of chips or cookies that are formulated to be compatible with this diet. Rather, you have to change how you think about food and be willing to make the necessary lifestyle changes to make whole, plant-based foods the centerpiece of your diet. These lifestyle changes include filling your shopping cart with produce rather than grains and meats, cooking meals at home (usually from scratch) instead of eating out, and eating food that is organic. The benefits produced by the plant-based diet — added years to life and life to years — make all of the effort worth it.

Chapter 9: Benefits of the Plant-Based Miracle Diet

Stabilize Blood Sugar and Blood Pressure

High blood sugar and high blood pressure are some of the biggest health woes causing disease today. However, the plant-based miracle diet can help stabilize and even reverse the conditions.

The elimination of all processed foods means that sugar consumption is drastically reduced; most sugars come from fruits and the breakdown of sprouted grains. As natural sources of sugar, these foods also contain high levels of fiber, which slows the sugar's absorption as well as the uptake of insulin. Because less sugar is entering the bloodstream, less insulin is needed to transport it to cells for energy. Even if someone already has developed insulin resistance, meaning that increasingly high levels of insulin are required to process the sugar, consuming less sugar means that less insulin will be required. Less sugar entering the blood, coupled with that sugar being processed efficiently by insulin so that it can be used by the cells, means that excess blood sugar is completely eradicated. Over time, stabilized blood sugar can lead to insulin resistance being reversed.

Sugar is a highly addictive substance, even more addictive than some illegal drugs. For the first few weeks, you may feel the effects of sugar withdrawal, which can include headaches, lightheadedness, anxiety, depression, moodiness, and irritability. You may be tempted to say that your blood sugar is too low and you need to eat a dessert to bring it back up. However, added sugars have absolutely no health benefit. Instead, you should eat fruit (a well-made fruit salad can satisfy a sweet tooth) and sprouted grains, which will keep your blood sugar stabilized instead of causing it to spike and then plummet.

In addition to helping stabilize your blood sugar, the plant-based miracle diet can help stabilize high blood pressure. The main culprits behind high blood pressure are obesity, which causes the heart to work harder, and processed food, which contains the bad fats, sugar, and salt that lead to heart disease. Eliminating processed foods can have almost immediate effects on blood pressure; a plant-based diet can lower it by up to 30% in weeks. Because a plant-based diet naturally leads to weight loss, it causes the heart to work less hard but more efficiently, thereby also lowering blood pressure.

Other Benefits

People who eat a plant-based diet have significantly lower rates of obesity; in fact, the plant-based miracle diet is the single most effective way of losing weight and keeping it off. As previously mentioned, obesity is linked to many health problems, including heart and cardiovascular disease, type 2 diabetes, metabolic syndrome, and high levels of stress. While in the 20th century and earlier most disease was due to starvation and malnourishment, obesity-related diseases are actually the product of a combination of overnutrition (too many calories) and malnutrition (not enough vitamins, minerals, and fiber).

When fiber intake is increased and the body is getting (and absorbing) enough nutrients, the excess weight begins to melt off. With reduced levels of sugar, hormones such as insulin become stabilized. Hormonal diseases, such as metabolic syndrome, insulin resistance, and type 2 diabetes, start to reverse. The wall of the gut begins to heal itself and the microbiome becomes healthy, causing problems such as autoimmune diseases and IBS to disappear without any medicinal intervention. The mood elevates, alleviating or even eliminating psychological problems such as depression and anxiety. Hardened arterial walls begin to soften, causing blood pressure to lower and thereby reducing the risk of stroke and other heart diseases. Without trans fats and bad cholesterol, arterial blockages are reduced and even eliminated, allowing for blood to flow freely throughout the body.

In summary, the benefits of the plant-based diet simply cannot be overstated. One of its most immediate effects is that high levels of blood sugar and high blood pressure begin to drop and reach safe, stable levels. In addition, it allows the body to heal itself so that other diseases and health problems, such as high cholesterol, obesity, and autoimmune diseases, are able to resolve themselves.

Chapter 10: Other Options and Diet

The Atkins Diet

The Atkins Diet took the United States by storm in the late 1990s and early 2000s. Dr. Robert C. Atkins promoted the diet and wrote a book about it in 1972. The theory behind it is that carbs are the reason we gain weight, so limiting carbs as much as possible leads to weight loss. People on the diet are advised to restrict consumption of any starchy or sugary foods, such as potatoes, bananas, wheat, apples, juice, and candy. The payoff is that they can eat as much protein (meat) and good fat as they want.

When Dr. Atkins began advocating this approach in the second half of the twentieth century, nutritionists and doctors were aghast. Fat was believed to be the enemy, and sugar was, for the most part, harmless (sugary processed foods like Snack Wells became popular during the 1980s and 1990s as diet foods). However, our understanding of nutrition has changed; we now understand that sugar is far worse, and fat in natural forms, such as olive oil and the fat in avocados, can actually be beneficial. Artificial fats, such as hydrogenated oils and trans fats, are to be avoided. Many people have boasted of being able to successfully lose weight on the Atkins diet. Proponents claim that it increases energy levels and actually reduces the risk of heart disease.

Unfortunately, the Atkins diet does not advocate exercise, claiming that it is not necessary for weight loss. Furthermore, the severely reduced consumption of carbs actually leads to eating fewer vegetables and almost no fruits, causing your body to not get the nutrients that it needs. Atkins is actually an animal-based diet.

The South Beach Diet

As the Atkins diet craze began to subside, the new South Beach diet began to rise in popularity. Its appeal over the Atkins diet was that it allowed for carbs to be incorporated. The push of the South Beach diet is the glycemic index, which determines whether particular carbs are good or bad. The glycemic index is a measure of how much and how quickly particular carbs will raise your blood sugar; whole grains are encouraged because they have a low glycemic index, while refined carbs and sugar are restricted because they have a high glycemic index. The South Beach diet promotes consumption of lean protein, whole grains, good fats, and fruits and vegetables.

One benefit of the South Beach diet is that it is more sustainable than the Atkins diet. The sheer amount of meat consumed on the Atkins diet is so high that on a global level, it is not environmentally sustainable. On a personal level, it can become very expensive, very quickly. Because the South Beach diet advocates a moderate intake of low-fat meat, such as chicken and fish, it is more environmentally and personally feasible. More people are able to follow it long-term because it allows for a moderate consumption of carbs. The higher intake of fruits and vegetables, over the Atkins diet, means that people on the South Beach diet are getting more nutrients. However, as you have previously read, the consumption of whole grains means more lectins, which lead to leaky gut syndrome.

The Paleo Diet

One of the latest diets to hit the US is the so-called paleo diet. The premise of the paleo diet is that our bodies evolved to process certain foods, the ones that our paleolithic ancestors ate. These foods included fruits and vegetables, lean meats, nuts and seeds, and fish. Modern farming began approximately 10,000 years ago; foods associated with modern farming are not compatible with the way that our bodies evolved. These foods include dairy, grains, and legumes. Modern processed foods and any added sugar are absolutely avoided.

The paleo diet has proven to be more beneficial than the Atkins or South Beach diets. Benefits of the paleo diet include decreased leptins, especially since grains and legumes are eliminated. It naturally includes a higher amount of fruits and vegetables to compensate for the lack of grains. Because our paleolithic ancestors were always active, the paleo diet advocates exercise every day; exercise has proven to be beneficial to both physical and emotional health. Even though the paleo diet is not a weight-loss formula, advocates say that they lose weight on it. They also have increased glucose tolerance, lower levels of triglycerides, and a stabilized appetite. However, the paleo diet does not address the problem of lectins.

Why the Plant-Based Diet is Best

The plant-based diet is the best of all of these other diet plans because, rather than being primarily a means to lose weight, it addresses the root causes of disease and advocates a healthy lifestyle. Reducing consumption of meat is shown to reduce blood pressure; eliminating it completely reduces it even more. In addition, raising animals for meat consumes far more environmental resources than growing the plants that underlie the plant-based diet. The plant-based diet addresses critical areas, such as the microbiome and lining of the intestines that are ignored by even the paleo diet. The plant-based diet is better for humans and for the environment.

In summary, the plant-based diet is not a fad or a means for quick weight loss. While weight loss is a result, that is merely a side benefit. Its goal is overall health and well-being. In addition to being better for your own personal health, the plant-based diet is better for the environment.

Chapter 11: Myths and Dangers

The world of health food and diets has become so commercialized that any diet comes with a host of critics and advocates, and along with them, seemingly contradictory information. If you do a Google search for veganism, vegetarianism, Atkins diet, plant-based diet, lectins, or any number of terms associated with healthy eating, you will receive so many different accounts, based on different information, that you may be tempted to forego healthy eating altogether. Knowing what to feed our bodies for optimal health and well-being seems to be the insurmountable task. There are some myths associated with the plant-based miracle diet, which this chapter will explain and dispel. It will also highlight some of the dangers of a plant-based diet, with the purpose of giving you the information you need to overcome them.

Myth 1: Whole grains and dairy are important sources of vital nutrients.

Despite the growing prevalence of leaky gut syndrome and increasing evidence that it is correlated with, if not caused by, dairy and the lectins found in whole grains, many nutritionists insist that both are necessary components of a healthy diet because of the nutrients found in them. However, there are no nutrients found in whole grains and dairy that can't be found elsewhere. Green, leafy vegetables, such as broccoli, kale, spinach, and parsley, are high in the B vitamins commonly found in whole grains but without the high level of lectins, as well as the calcium touted by dairy. Consuming these foods will not only reduce the amount of lectin you ingest and therefore help heal your intestinal lining but will also increase the prebiotics that feed your gut's microbiome.

Myth 2: Animal protein is superior to plant protein.

Other primates, including gorillas, have muscles that are far bigger than ours. However, they derive virtually all of their protein from plant sources. The fact is that amino acids are created by plants, which are then consumed by animals. Animals create some amino acids, but these can be obtained from plants. In fact, all plants contain all nine essential amino acids; therefore, consuming a sufficient amount of plant-based food will ensure that you get enough protein. The rule of thumb is that if you are getting enough calories from a plant-based diet, then you are getting enough protein.

Myth 3: A plant-based diet is prohibitively expensive.

Healthier food is certainly more expensive, especially when placed side-by-side with its processed counterparts. If a loaf of white bread costs one dollar and a loaf of sprouted-grain bread costs five dollars, one can easily conclude that healthy food is five times more expensive. However, that is only part of the actual situation.

Most Americans go out to eat between three and five times per week. If the average cost of a restaurant meal is ten dollars, then that is as much as fifty dollars a week going to unhealthy restaurant food! If you put that much money towards buying plant-based food rather than convenient restaurant food, you will probably end up spending about the same amount.

Many people on a plant-based diet report that they actually spend less on food than they previously did when eating a diet high in animal products and grains. Furthermore, they spend less on health-related issues, making the savings even more.

Myth 4: B12 is only found in meat.

Vitamin B12 is actually created by bacteria, not by animals. Animal products contain B12 because the bacteria in the animals create the B12. Properly fermented vegetable-based foods, such as natto (fermented soy), can be used to meet a person's B12 needs.

Danger 1: Plants don't contain Vitamin A in the form that our bodies need.

Our bodies need Vitamin A in the form of retinol, but what plants give us is beta-carotene, which is then converted into retinol. Based on conditions such as the health of your gut, your thyroid function, and some genetic factors, your body's ability to convert beta-carotene into retinol could be compromised. In order to avoid this danger, take the necessary steps to ensure that your gut is properly functioning so that it can properly convert beta-carotene into retinol. You may want to get a periodic blood test to ensure that you have appropriate levels of Vitamin A.

Danger 2: Not consuming animal products can reduce the amount of stomach acid, thereby reducing the overall efficiency of the digestive system.

When you consume animal products, especially meat, your stomach creates more hydrochloric acid (stomach acid) to assist in the breakdown of proteins. The digestive process is driven largely by a balanced pH, meaning that stomach acid is necessary to kick-start digestion. Without adequate stomach acid, the body is actually less able to absorb the nutrients that you consume. This condition is called hypochlorhydria. It results in abdominal discomfort, bloating, and gas immediately after eating and can lead to malnutrition from lack of nutrient absorption.

In order to prevent hypochlorhydria, drink a cup of room-temperature water with a tablespoon of apple cider vinegar before meals. The apple cider vinegar will help stimulate the stomach to produce the necessary acid.

Also, keep in mind that digestion is not merely a physical process. It is actually a parasympathetic process that involves both the mind and the body. Emotional distress can actually impede digestion. Maintaining a stress-free lifestyle and being relaxed when you eat can also combat hypochlorhydria.

In summary, many of the reasons why people decide not to follow the plant-based diet are based on faulty logic and science. There are no nutrients found in animal sources that cannot also be derived from plants, and usually with higher quality. While there are potential dangers in following the plant-based diet, they can be alleviated by taking simple measures.

Chapter 12: The Importance of Nutrition

Even though Dr. Atkins claimed that exercise is not necessary for weight loss, it is a necessary aspect of overall health and well-being. Eighty percent of wellness is based on diet, while the other twenty percent is based on exercise. This chapter will look at that concept in more detail.

Eighty Percent Diet

It goes without saying that the food you eat is incredibly important. Proper nutrition can prevent many of the diseases associated with modern society and reverse them in people who already have them. This section will look at some important vitamins and minerals and give you information on what they do and what plant-based foods contain them.

Iron is a mineral usually obtained from red meat, but it is also present in green leafy vegetables, such as kale, spinach, and broccoli, as well as eggs and shellfish. It is required by red blood cells in order for them to transport oxygen throughout the body. Iron deficiency is known as anemia; it causes cells throughout the body to become hypoxic (lacking in oxygen). As a result, someone with anemia will feel weak, fatigued, and may even faint.

Vitamin D has gained a lot of popularity in the health community over the past few years, and for good reason. Its functions include allowing the body to absorb calcium, which is necessary for bone health, regulating the immune system so that it functions properly, and protecting against cancer. Low levels of vitamin D are linked with many different cancers, weight gain, heart disease, and depression. It can be obtained from egg yolks and wild fish, but the body actually produces it naturally from sunlight. In order to have optimum levels of vitamin D, the best thing to do is get plenty of sunshine.

Vitamin K is an unsung hero, as vitamin D has attracted so much attention. Vitamin K allows the blood to clot and aids in the transportation of calcium throughout the body, making it essential for healing injuries and protecting bone health. Without vitamin K, a simple wound can lead to so much blood flow that the injured person can resemble a hemophiliac. This important nutrient can be found in pretty much any fruit or vegetable that is green: Brussels sprouts, spinach, kiwi, avocado, broccoli, cabbage, kale, chard, and grapes.

Vitamin B1, or thiamine, is required by the body in order to process carbohydrates and proteins. Many people rely on whole grains to obtain thiamine, but it can also be found in nuts and some vegetables, such as peas.

Vitamin B2, or riboflavin, aids in the production of red blood cells and converting food into energy. Without an adequate supply of B2, no matter how many calories you consume, you will still feel lethargic. It can be obtained by eating almonds and asparagus and is also found in dark chicken meat.

Vitamin B6 is crucial because, like B2, it helps convert food into energy; it also aids in the breakdown of sugar, making it particularly beneficial for people who have developed insulin resistance or type 2 diabetes. It can be found in peas, spinach, and bananas; those who choose to consume small amounts of animal products can also find it in light poultry meat and eggs.

Vitamin C is touted for its ability to help boost people's immune systems. More than that, it is critical for the formation of collagen (the main protein found in the connective tissue between cells) and in creating some of the chemical messengers that the brain uses to transport its electrical signals. Sugary processed foods, such as gummy fruit snacks, and sugary juices like to boast of containing high levels of vitamin C; however, more than ample amounts of it can be found in nearly any fruit. Instead of drinking a glass of orange juice to help fight off a cold, eat a whole orange. You will get plenty of vitamin C that has not been subjected to the processing required to make orange juice; the whole orange will also provide you with the fiber needed to prevent a spike in blood sugar.

Vitamin E is a powerful antioxidant that protects cells from damage that can be incurred from toxins and the normal aging process. It is also important for skin health; medical professionals may apply pure vitamin E directly to a severe skin injury. It can be found in plant-based foods that are high in fat, such as olive oil, avocados, and nuts. Keep in mind that while some oils, such as corn, soy, canola, and vegetable oil, are also derived from plants, they are created in laboratories and are full of damaging trans fats. They should be avoided as often as possible.

Folate is particularly important for pregnant women because it helps prevent birth defects. It also aids in heart health and in the creation of red blood cells. Many people rely on grains, beans, and lentils to obtain it, but it can be found in plentiful supply in dark green vegetables.

Calcium is important for healthy bone growth and development, as well as for transporting messages between cells and helping muscles work. Its benefits are widely touted as part of a campaign to get Americans to drink more milk; however, milk contributes to leaky gut syndrome. Furthermore, the calcium found in milk is not the best kind. The best calcium can be found in broccoli and dark leafy vegetables. For those who opt to consume animal products, it is also found in fish and fish bones (which are edible).

Magnesium is another unsung hero in the arsenal of vitamins and minerals. It improves nerve function, decreases anxiety, improves sleep, alleviates muscle pain, improves heart health, prevents migraines, and relieves constipation. This vital mineral can be found in dark leafy greens, nuts, avocados, and bananas. It can also be obtained by taking a bath with Epsom salt.

Zinc helps boost immune function so that you can heal faster. It strengthens the hair, skin, and nails, and a plentiful supply of zinc can even diminish scars! Many Americans obtain zinc through red meat and poultry, but it can also be found in nuts and seafood. Zinc supplements can also be beneficial but are no substitute for a good diet.

Twenty Percent Exercise

If twenty percent of health and well-being is dependent on exercise, then without it, even the most nutritious diet in the world will only bring eighty percent of your health potential. The twenty-percent deficit could leave you prone to depression, anxiety, and physiological disease. This section will look at different types of exercise and the benefits that they can produce.

Cardio exercise is basically any exercise that raises the heart rate. It includes brisk walking, running, swimming, stair stepping, bike riding, rowing, and dancing, amongst other things. Cardio exercise produces many benefits, beginning with promoting heart health. Muscles are healthier when they are used, and the heart is no exception. Elevating the heart rate during 30-minute to hour-and-a-half sessions of cardio workouts can strengthen the heart so that it actually creates more capillaries, thereby allowing blood to flow more freely throughout the body. It also burns off unwelcome substances that can build up in the blood and other parts of the body, such as triglycerides, excess sugar, and stress hormones. As a result, it leads to weight loss, increased energy, elevated mood, and decreased stress. Whatever your exercise routine may be, you should make time for at least thirty minutes of cardio most days of the week.

Strength exercises help to keep your bones and muscles strong. They include lifting weights and resistance training, such as using resistance bands or resistance machines. Strength exercise is not just for the young; older people in particular benefit from it because it helps them maintain their independence and prevent falls.

Flexibility exercises help maintain a wide range of motion while keeping your body limber. The range of motion refers to the extent to which you are able to move different parts of your body; people with conditions such as bursitis can benefit from flexibility exercises, as they can help extend the range of motion and thereby help the person get back his or her abilities. Flexibility exercises include doing yoga and stretching various parts of the body.

Balance exercises, such as tai chi, standing on one foot, some yoga positions, and heel-to-toe walking, help to strengthen the body's core. A stronger core promotes overall health, especially digestive and gut health, and decreases the risk of diseases that begin in the abdomen (such as type 2 diabetes and some autoimmune diseases).

In summary, the plant-based diet is able to provide you with all of the nutrients necessary to achieve optimal functioning of the entire body. Even nutrients typically obtained from meat, such as iron.

Chapter 13: Safety, Side Effects, and Warnings

Despite its superior benefits, the plant-based miracle diet does not come without some of its vices. These vices, however, do not outweigh the benefits of the diet.

Many Americans are incredibly deficient in fiber; while 97% of Americans get enough protein (because of all the meat that they consume), 97% of Americans do not get enough fiber. The average fiber intake is only fifteen grams per day, while the body needs 32 grams per day! Switching to a plant-based diet means a significantly higher intake of fiber, which may take some adjusting. Common side effects of increased fiber intake include bloating, abdominal cramps, gas, and diarrhea. Less common side effects include temporary weight gain (usually from water) and constipation. In order to mitigate these side effects, make the switch to the plant-based diet gradually. Instead of immediately jumping from one or two servings of fruits and vegetables per day to ten, build that number up over the course of a few weeks. Not only will this allow your system to adjust, but it will also give you time to adjust your lifestyle to accommodate the plant-based diet.

One benefit of the plant-based diet is that it cleanses toxins that have accumulated in your body from years of unhealthy eating. Some people immediately feel great. However, for some people, this purge can lead to symptoms of detox, including aches and pains, fatigue, irritability, and other ailments commonly associated with the flu. Most Americans are addicted to sugar; sugar has actually hijacked their brains similar to narcotics and other addictive substances so that the brain is tricked into thinking that it has to have it. Switching to the plant-based diet may involve a withdrawal process, which can include anxiety, depression, intense cravings, moodiness, and brain fog. In order to mitigate these side effects, eat fruit whenever a sugar craving hits. Drinking a calming beverage, such as lemon balm tea, throughout the day can help lessen the anxiety and moodiness.

Consider the transition process, in which your body adjusts to the plant-based diet, as any transition process. Transitions are not ever easy. Think of it like getting a new puppy. The new puppy is cute, playful, and cuddly, so much so that you would not dream of getting rid of it. However, that puppy has to be house trained so as to not constantly do its business on the floor (or any other unwelcome place). This process involves completely changing your routine so that you are available every few hours to take the puppy outside. Furthermore, the puppy wants to chew on everything, including your expensive shoes. You have to learn to put all of your things away so that the puppy cannot chew on them, and will still have to replace some things that were important. However, as your routine adjusts to life with a puppy, you grow fond of it as it contributes to increasing your own happiness and quality of life. You love playing with it, and seeing it happy makes you happy. One day, you will look back on those days of adjustment to life with a puppy with fondness and won't even think about all the potty accidents or chewed-up shoes.

Likewise, when you make the transition to a plant-based diet, the process may be hard and require some serious adjusting. However, once your body gets used to it, you will feel so good and will have such an increased quality of life that you won't have any desire to go back.

Some people wonder whether the plant-based diet is for them. Simply put, the plant-based diet is for everyone. People of all ages and at all stages of life can benefit from it. Pregnant women who plan their meals appropriately can benefit immensely from the plant-based diet. It can counteract some of the fatigue and morning sickness brought on by pregnancy while still providing the developing baby with all of the nutrients necessary to thrive. In addition, pregnant women on the plant-based diet have a markedly lower chance of developing gestational diabetes and other pregnancy complications.

Children, even infants, can benefit from the plant-based diet. While infants need high levels of fat, this can be obtained from the mother's breast milk. Following the World Health Organization guidelines of breastfeeding for two years will ensure that your child will get all of the fat needed throughout the infant and toddler years. Children raised on the plant-based diet have fewer behavioral problems, including ADD and ADHD.

Athletes and bodybuilders are notorious for consuming large quantities of meat and other animal products in order to fuel their muscles for intense training sessions. However, they can get all of the nutrients that they need on a plant-based diet, especially one that calls for eating free-range, grass-fed meat once or twice a week. All of the nutrients needed for cellular and muscular growth and repair can be found in plants; small amounts of meat and other animal products can work as a supplement.

In summary, there are some drawbacks to the plant-based diet, but nothing that cannot be overcome. The uncomfortable effects of a drastic increase in fiber intake can be mitigated by gradually increasing the amount of fiber in the diet until optimal levels are achieved. The symptoms of detox that come from flushing the toxins from the body can be very uncomfortable, but again, a gradual transition can ease this process. Withdrawal from sugar addiction can be the hardest part of the transition for some people; to help get through it, eat a lot of fruit and drink herbal tea.

Chapter 14: The Light Dieters

Light dieters are individuals who want the benefits of the plant-based diet but are unable to make a commitment for a total change. They change one meal a day and aim to make the other two meals as healthy as possible. This chapter is specifically for people whose lifestyles may be inflexible due to occupational, financial, or any other reasons. Construction workers, athletes, shift workers, and others who need a lot of energy and are not able to take the time to deal with the side effects of going entirely plant-based are ideal candidates. People who want to experiment with the plant-based diet to see if it is something they can stick with are also ideal candidates. This regimen also applies to people who want to change to eating entirely a plant-based diet but are making the change gradually.

Changing One Meal a Day

Changing one meal a day from being meat-based to being plant-based is one way to substantially benefit your own health as well as the health of the planet. If every American switched one meal a week from being meat-based to being entirely vegan, the environmental equivalent would be like taking half a million cars off the road! To further increase the benefit both to your own health, the local economy, and the global environment make that one meal per day locally sourced from small farmers in your area.

The immediate benefits of changing one meal a day to being plant-based include that your daily servings of fruits and vegetables will go up. Many people rely on meat for their protein intake; however, some fruits and vegetables, such as jackfruit, are also high in protein as well as other vital vitamins and minerals. Choosing to use these plant-based sources of protein, even only one time each day, will provide the added benefit of extra fiber and other essential nutrients.

Your palate will expand as you try new fruits and vegetables that you previously had not even heard of. You may find that there are a lot of plant-based foods out there that you enjoy more than you did processed foods! This will encourage you to further increase your intake of a variety of fruits and vegetables and completely eliminate all processed foods. You may not even be tempted to go back to your old ways of eating.

Changing just one meal a day will allow you to gain many of the benefits of the plant-based diet, including improved overall health and vitality; reduction, reversal, and even elimination of chronic as well as acute diseases; and more energy. Furthermore, some of the unpleasant side effects — such as gas, bloating, diarrhea, and constipation — will be alleviated compared to those who make the full switch immediately. In other words, by changing just one meal a day to being completely plant-based, you should expect to feel better!

There is an important caveat, one known as the law of compensatory consumption. When we make positive changes, we tend to subconsciously justify doing more of our negative, detrimental habits because we feel so good about ourselves. For example, when people decide to use less water to help reduce their environmental footprints, they oftentimes subconsciously use more energy than they did previously; this is because they feel that their decreased water consumption justifies an increased use of electricity. People who switch to one plant-based meal a day will feel the temptation to eat more meat and processed foods at other meals. Be aware of this temptation so that you can resist it! Keep at the forefront of your mind the reason why you are making the switch to one plant-based meal per day so that you don't even want to eat more meat or processed foods. Don't fall prey to the law of compensatory consumption!

In summary, making the switch to eating one plant-based meal per day is a great way to kick off a lifestyle of healthy eating. You can begin to reap the benefits of the plant-based miracle diet but without many of the unpleasant side effects that can come with it. In addition, by making the change gradually, you are more likely to stick with the diet rather than if you jumped in all the way without giving yourself a transition period.

Chapter 15: Intermediate Dieters

Intermediate dieters are people who change two meals per day from being meat-based to being plant-based. Maybe they have already gone through the transition of changing one meal a day and can't get enough of the positive benefits. They want to continue making the switch to being entirely plant-based eaters. Other people who are ideal candidates for being intermediate dieters are those who have active social lives that include eating out with friends and/or family on a frequent basis. While restaurant meals almost inevitably contain animal products unless the menu says otherwise, eating a plant-based diet for two meals a day can compensate for the restaurant meals. In addition, busy moms whose families are resistant to eating a plant-based diet are ideal for changing two meals per day; they can eat a plant-based breakfast and lunch and then enjoy the same supper as their families. Meanwhile, all of the people making the switch to changing two meals a day from being meat-based to being plant-based are reaping even more of the rewards of the plant-based miracle diet.

Benefits, Expectations, and Results

The benefits of changing two meals per day from being meat-based to being plant-based are substantial. Most energy consumption in the sector of agriculture and food production comes from meat; it actually takes up to five times more water and a hundred times more food to produce a pound of meat as opposed to a pound of vegetables. The first benefit is a significantly reduced environmental impact. If the two plant-based meals that you eat each day are sourced from local small farmers and are organic (many small farmers use organic growing techniques, even if their produce is not certified as organic), the environmental impact is reduced even further. The second benefit is even more energy. While changing one meal a day to a plant-based diet increases energy levels substantially, changing two meals a day increases them even more. By giving your body the proper vitamins and minerals, as opposed to just the calories, that it needs, it is able to use the calories that it has consumed as energy. With that increased energy, you will *want* to exercise; rather than being a chore, exercise will become an indispensable part of your daily routine. Reaping all of the benefits of exercise is reason enough to make the change! Another benefit is increased alertness and improved mood. Brain fog, irritability, depression, and anxiety can all be caused, at least to an extent, by a poor diet that is high in processed foods and animal products. Eliminating processed foods and significantly reducing the number of animal products consumed can quickly turn those conditions around without any medication.

Just like with the one-meal-per-day switch, if you make the two-meal-per-day switch, you should expect to feel better. Your body will cleanse out more of the toxins that accumulated due to years of poor diet. While at first, you may experience some fatigue and withdrawal, especially if you didn't first make the transition to one plant-based meal per day, those effects are the result of your body being purged of all those toxins. After a few days, once your body has been cleansed, you will feel drastically better. Inflammation, and all of the problems that come with it — such as chronic aches and pains — will go down. Your gut will begin to heal, and its microbiome will be restored to optimal levels. In addition, excess weight will begin to fall off.

As with making the switch to one plant-based meal per day, make sure that you don't succumb to the law of compensatory consumption. Don't eat extra junk food to make up for all of the healthy food that you are now eating. If you must, splurge in another area. Get yourself a nice haircut or buy a new outfit to complement your now-healthy body. But don't steer off course! Then again, why would you even want to?

In summary, making the switch to eating two plant-based meals per day augments the benefits of eating one plant-based meal per day. Energy, vitality, and overall health and well-being are increased. The body flushes out the toxins that have accumulated and begins to heal itself, without the need for medication. The result is a happier and healthier you!

Chapter 16: Hard-Core Dieters

Hard-core dieting, in reference to the plant-based diet, is not an exercise in restriction or deprivation. Rather, it is a lifestyle of eating exclusively plant-based foods and reaping the benefits. While changing one or two meals a day is an ideal way for a lot of people to regain their health, especially people who are unwilling or unable to commit to an exclusively plant-based diet, going entirely vegan is for those who are completely committed to their health and well-being.

There are many lifestyle changes involved in eating nothing but the plant-based miracle diet. One of them is that socializing with friends will no longer involve going out to eat at any restaurant you or your friends should choose. Either the restaurant will have to have vegan options, or you will have to content yourself with watching everybody else eat. An alternative will be to invite friends over to your house for a vegan meal before going out on the town (or whatever you enjoy doing with your friends). An even better alternative is to not go solo when switching to the plant-based diet. See if any of your friends or family want to join in your endeavors. If no one wants to, at least try to earn the support of the people closest to you. That way, when you speak up about wanting to go to a restaurant that has vegan options, the people around you are more likely to acquiesce. They may even want to try vegan options, too!

Other lifestyle changes that you will probably encounter in the transition to full veganism include having to read food labels to determine if something is truly vegan and incorporating plant-based protein sources that aren't high in damaging lectins, such as natto. You will probably face some challenges in the transition, including the side effects mentioned in an earlier chapter. However, the benefits are life-changing.

People who went completely vegan for a mere 60 days reported that no matter how much they ate, they still lost weight. They experienced less soreness and had so much energy that they didn't know what to do with themselves. Six weeks in, they were prepared to make the transition permanent.

In summary, making the change to complete veganism is hard. It involves a lot of lifestyle changes and learning to eat in an entirely different way. However, it also leads to a revitalized body with exceptionally high energy levels.

Chapter 17: Going Organic

Dangers of Pesticide Use and Conventional Farming

In the year 1962, an American writer named Rachel Carson published a book entitled *Silent Spring*. The book highlighted how the use of heavy pesticides, including the supposedly safe one known as DDT, which was used commercially for agriculture and at home. The pesticide was known to cause cancer, yet was being sprayed indiscriminately into the environment. No long-term study had shown what its long-term environmental impact would be, but the bird population — including the emblematic bald eagle — was deteriorating because of its use. The title, *Silent Spring*, hearkened to the idea that with continued use of pesticides, we might experience a spring in which no birds sing. A public outcry ensued, which led to the banning of DDT in the year 1972.

Modern agricultural chemicals, however, may actually be worse than DDT. Glyphosate, the active ingredient in the commercially available pesticide Round-Up, was approved for use in 1974, shortly after the banning of DDT. Most bacteria are actually beneficial, especially those that comprise your gut's microbiome. Glyphosate actually kills most of the beneficial bacteria, both in the soil and in your gut. As a result, disease-causing bacteria are able to proliferate. It also damages the nutrients in the soil so that the plants are not able to properly absorb them, leading to sick plants and nutrient-deficient food. Glyphosate decreases the body's ability to detoxify foreign invaders and process organic compounds, further contributing to disease. Furthermore, it is toxic to human DNA, thereby holding the potential to devastate the entire human genome. It also disrupts the reproductive system, leading to problems such as infertility and birth defects.

Glyphosate has been linked with the rise of many diseases. For example, the rise in the use of glyphosate corresponds almost perfectly with the rise in autism spectrum disorder in children. It is a known carcinogen, meaning that it causes cancer, and may also be linked to Alzheimer's.

The environmental impact of glyphosate is unprecedented. It has built up in soils, damaging local micro-ecosystems. In fact, it has penetrated so deeply into the soil that it is contaminating water in the underground water table. Rainfall naturally causes glyphosate to runoff into streams and rivers, where it wreaks havoc on marine life. Fish are showing genetic abnormalities. Male fish are showing female characteristics, and some are even dying out. From rivers and streams, glyphosate makes its way into the ocean, where it continues its path of destruction. While Monsanto, the company that manufactures glyphosate, claims that it disintegrates rapidly, its residues can be detected in water two weeks to well over a month after exposure. In soil, it can be detected six months or longer after exposure.

Glyphosate is not even the worst chemical used commercially today. 2,4-D is the active ingredient herbicide found in many weed killers that can be bought at a store. Commercial farmers and local households use it to kill weeds. However, 2,4-D comprised about half of the chemical known as Agent Orange, which was sprayed indiscriminately in the jungles of Vietnam to help soldiers navigate them during the war. Agent Orange caused diseases in approximately one-quarter of the people exposed to it, including birth defects, genetic mutations, and cancer. The chemical that you may be using to spray your own yard to kill weeds may be one of the two ingredients that composed Agent Orange!

GMOs

In 1994, the Flavr Savr tomato, the first genetically modified food, was approved for commercial distribution and sale. Since then, GMOs, or genetically modified organisms, have proliferated to such a degree that unless explicitly labeled otherwise, you can be almost certain that what you are eating was genetically modified. Not only are plants genetically modified, but some animals are, as well. In fact, the first documented case of successful genetic modification was a mouse, in 1973. Today, genetically modified salmon are sold at supermarkets across the country. Genetically modified fish, known as GloFish and adored for their vibrant colors, are sold as pets. Genetically modified mosquitoes have been released into the wild to combat malaria and other mosquito-borne diseases.

Genetic modification is usually done to create some purported benefit. For example, some bananas have been genetically modified to help increase the body's ability to process vitamin A, and other crops have been genetically modified to make them drought resistant. The process of genetic modification involves isolating a particular desired gene, such as one that enables a crop to survive with less water, and inserting it into the genome of the candidate plant's seeds. This artificial manipulation creates plants that actually don't exist in nature. In addition, the benefit that the GMO plant is supposed to bring just doesn't come. Supposedly drought-resistant GMO crops are not able to withstand water shortages; in fact, they tend to do poorer than their non-GMO counterparts.

Eighty percent of GMO crops around the world are genetically modified to be resistant to herbicides and pesticides, especially the dangerous pesticide glyphosate. In fact, the company that creates most GMO seeds, Monsanto, is the same company that produces Round-Up! Crops that are genetically modified to withstand high levels of glyphosate are termed "Roundup Ready," and are specifically cultivated to be sprayed with glyphosate. Estimates are that approximately 300 million pounds of Roundup are sprayed every year globally. With the known and documented effects of Roundup on both human and environmental health, one can only shudder at what its extensive use is doing. In response, the weeds that Round-Up is supposed to be killing, while preserving the crop plants, are actually developing resistance to the herbicide, meaning that higher and higher levels of it are required.

GMO food poses a double threat to humans. The first is that the altered DNA actually changes the DNA of the bacteria in the microbiome, making them unable to perform their functions, and even changes the DNA in some of your body's cells. It is actually disrupting the human genome! The second is that it is loaded with glyphosate, exposing you to higher and higher levels of this toxic chemical. That apple that you think is a healthy snack, unless labeled as being organic or non-GMO, could actually cause infertility, cancer, hormonal disruptions, and genetic mutations!

Benefits of Organic Farming Techniques

As opposed to conventional, large agriculture, which relies heavily on the use of agrichemicals and leads to problems such as soil degradation and wasted water, organic farming uses techniques that are beneficial to the environment. Instead of artificial fertilizers, organic farming uses natural fertilizers, such as manure and compost. Instead of dangerous chemicals, it uses pesticides that are naturally created by plants or even insects, such as ladybugs. To keep the soil fertile, crop rotation is used. Instead of working against the environment by using artificial means to grow crops, it works with the environment by utilizing natural forces to produce a chemical-free crop.

Benefits of Eating Organic Food

The benefits of eating organic food over conventionally grown food are tremendous. People who switch to organic food routinely find that problems such as food allergies completely disappear. This could be because modern farming techniques, especially the cultivation of genetically modified food, is creating food sensitivities and allergies in otherwise healthy people. Another benefit is that people who eat organic food have substantially lower levels of chemical residue in their bodies. Therefore, they experience fewer of the health problems associated with high herbicide and pesticide use. In addition, because chemical toxins are often stored in fat cells, reducing those toxins can actually allow you to lose weight without necessarily reducing calorie intake! Because organic food is grown in healthier soil that retains its nutrients, it can even have a higher nutrient content than its conventional counterpart. All in all, organic food is better for you and for the environment.

In summary, modern, conventional farming techniques are devastating the health of the human population and of the planet. Heavy chemical use is damaging entire ecosystems, and GMO foods are causing even more extensive damage. However, organic farming techniques and the consumption of organic food hold great potential for reversing both environmental and human health problems.

Chapter 18: Complement to a Healthier You

The Ketogenic Diet

Our long-ago ancestors did not eat three meals a day, like we do. They hunted and foraged for food, and if there was no food, they simply didn't eat. However, in most cases, they didn't starve. Rather, their bodies adapted to this lifestyle by burning off fat as a primary energy source rather than sugar. In modern society, sugar is the most-used energy source, so much so that traditional nutritional wisdom says that glucose (a type of sugar) is the body's primary energy source. This reinforces the false idea that we need to eat a lot of carbs. Our bodies are actually very capable of using fat as a primary energy source; in fact, from a metabolic perspective, fat is a more stable and sustainable form of energy than sugar.

Ketones are substances created by the liver when it breaks down fat, thereby creating energy. Ketones are also important for brain health and mental function, so getting the body to create more ketones improves both the mind and body. The diet actually was developed as a way of treating neurological disorders! Most of the time, our bodies primarily rely on glucose, a simple form of sugar derived from carbs, as energy. As a result, the fat that is stored in our bodies is not burned; therefore, we are unable to lose weight. The ketogenic diet is about significantly reducing the amount of carbs eaten so that the body begins to burn fat liver produces the ketones to generate energy. Starving the body of carbs forces it into a metabolic state known as ketosis, which literally means that ketones are being broken down.

On the ketogenic diet, carbs only account for five to ten percent of all calories consumed, and those carbs come exclusively from fruits and vegetables. Seventy-five percent of all calories come from fat, and the remaining ones come from protein. The high-fat content is crucial to establishing an optimal state of ketosis; a high-fat diet also decreases hunger and appetite, as well as cravings for carbs. The fats should come from healthy, natural sources, such as avocados, unprocessed cheese, nuts, eggs, and red meat. The protein is derived from these high-fat foods. Variations on the ketogenic diet include cycling, with five days on and two days of high-carb intake, higher protein intake (suitable for athletes and bodybuilders), and adding in carbs around your workout schedule.

Because the body's own fat stores are being used for energy, the ketogenic diet quickly leads to weight loss. In addition, it has many other benefits, as well. The extremely low intake of carbs leads to greater mental clarity and performance, leading to increased productivity. Without insulin being generated to aid in the transportation of glucose, people on the ketogenic diet become more energetic and have a more regulated sense of being hungry and full. Lower, stabilized insulin can reverse the effects of insulin resistance and even type 2 diabetes. People with acne tend to benefit from the ketogenic diet as well, as it helps lead to clearer skin. Despite the high amount of fats consumed, it actually lowers cholesterol and blood pressure. In addition, the ketogenic diet has been the primary method of treating children with epilepsy for over a hundred years. It reduces the amount of medication that they have to take and leads to better outcomes. The ketogenic diet is also believed to reduce the risk, symptoms, and progression of Alzheimer's disease and aid in recovery from brain trauma.

The ketogenic diet has been shown to improve insulin levels in people who are diabetic and prediabetic, thereby alleviating the symptoms and even the disease. However, people who are diabetic should only go on the ketogenic diet under a doctor's supervision. Inability to create insulin means that glucose is unable to enter the cells to be used as energy, so the liver burns fats to create higher and higher levels of ketones. This can lead to a condition called ketoacidosis, which causes the body's pH to become so acidic that it can be fatal. Someone who does not have diabetes is at an immeasurably low risk of developing ketoacidosis; it usually only occurs in individuals whose diabetes is unmanaged.

Intermittent Fasting

Intermittent fasting is the process of starving the body of all calories so that it is forced into a metabolic state in which body fat is quickly burned and muscle is easily built. The idea behind it is that what you eat is not as important as when you eat; therefore, you don't have to give up any of the foods that you enjoy. Instead, you should only eat at certain times.

When food is consumed, the body spends about five hours digesting it; during digestion, hormones that lead to weight gain, especially insulin, are activated. Because most people eat within five hours of their last meal or snack, they are unable to enter into the stage in which they can lose weight because the fat-storing, weight-gaining hormones are constantly coursing through them. Intentionally foregoing meals by going through periods of fasting and feeding put the body into a state in which body fat is burned. You can drink as much water and calorie-free beverages (such as green tea and coffee) as you want but only eat at certain times. Fasting times usually range from 12 to 20 hours, but some programs have fasting periods that last as long as 36 hours.

The idea of intermittent fasting goes against traditional nutritional advice, which says that in order to keep the metabolism moving, you need to eat small meals all throughout the day. Eating small meals leads to a higher metabolic rate, while foregoing food puts the body into starvation mode, causing the metabolism to slow down and fat to be stockpiled. The problem with this traditional wisdom is that it is built on the idea that glucose, rather than fat, should be the body's primary energy source. In order for the body to continually provide energy through glucose, there does need to be a constant supply of food. However, that glucose raises insulin levels, leading to weight gain, not weight loss. The wisdom of intermittent fasting is that it relies on lowering insulin levels so that the body burns fat with little effort.

There are several different intermittent fasting programs, including LeanGains, the Warrior Diet, Fat Loss Forever, the Alternate

Day Diet, and Eat Stop Eat. The Warrior Diet was one of the first diets to bring in the idea of intermittent fasting. It is based on the concept that in ancient civilizations (and even sometimes in modern ones), warriors or soldiers did not stop during the day to eat. Rather, they marched, trained, and battled during the day and only ate in the evenings. However, they were fit, alert, and capable of facing the enemy. On the Warrior Diet, you fast for 20 hours every day and consume all of your daily nutritional needs within a four-hour feeding window in the evenings. This regimen can be difficult to adopt all at once, so people on the Warrior Diet usually transition into it gradually. LeanGains is an intermittent fasting plan that incorporates workouts into the fasting and feeding schedule so as to optimize fat burn and muscle build. Other intermittent fasting plans, such as Fat Loss Forever and the Alternate Day Diet, use various schedules of feeding, fasting, and workouts so as to get the best results.

The benefits of intermittent fasting go beyond weight loss; it also helps improve cardiovascular health, energy levels, and mental clarity. Adjusting to intermittent fasting can be challenging, especially because until the body fully adjusts, periods of fasting can involve intense hunger, irritability, anxiety, and moodiness. Given time, the body is usually able to adjust quite well so as to reap the benefits of intermittent fasting. Some religious groups already advocate intermittent fasting, such as Muslims who fast during Ramadan. If fasting is already a part of your spiritual life, then intermittent fasting can be a way to kill two birds with one stone; you can get both the physical and spiritual benefits.

Many people can benefit from intermittent fasting. Those who have been trying to lose those last five or ten pounds, people who enjoy working out frequently, and people who already fast for reasons other than weight loss can benefit from implementing an intermittent fasting regimen. Pregnant women and people with certain diseases, including diabetes and ones that require a ketogenic diet (as opposed to being on a ketogenic diet voluntarily), should not try intermittent fasting. Additionally, some people have difficult schedules that can make intermittent fasting difficult, if not impossible. College students, shift workers, and people who must be on-call for work may have a very difficult time adapting an intermittent fasting program into their lifestyles. They may want to try another health and wellness program, such as the plant-based miracle diet or the ketogenic diet.

For more information, you can check out my book on intermittent fasting.

Exercise

The benefits of exercise are well-known and documented. People who exercise regularly experience lower levels of disease, higher levels of energy, a more moderated appetite, and higher overall health and well-being. Many people have been able to get off of a variety of medicines, everything from antidepressants to statins, because exercise alone was enough to alleviate the symptoms and even cure the underlying cause of illness. In order to get the most out of exercise, you need to get your heart rate above normal. While adding casual walks into your daily routine is beneficial in many ways, vigorous exercise that gets the heart pumping and forces you to breathe harder is the best. A brisk morning walk, taking the stairs at work, and a trip to the gym are all great ways to add heart-healthy exercise into your daily regimen.

Accountability Partners

Accountability partners are an important component of staying on track as you make the lifestyle changes necessary to become healthier. Your accountability partner may be someone who is more of a mentor that has already gone through the process; this mentorship set-up has shown to have great results in programs like Alcoholics Anonymous. Your accountability partner may also be a friend or peer who, like you, wants to get healthy. People who have accountability partners are much more successful at reaching their overall goals.

The key to having an effective accountability partnership is easy: Stay accountable to each other! Plan to connect with each other at least once a week to share how that week has been going. Did you fall off the wagon and into the sugar trap? Did you have a meat craving that you just couldn't ignore? How does your accountability partner deal with cravings? What are some of the benefits that you are seeing from your lifestyle changes? An accountability partner can give you an extra layer of vision that you don't have on your own because he or she can see things that you cannot. For example, you may see that the numbers on the scale haven't budged, but your accountability partner may notice that you look slimmer and your skin is brighter. He or she can also give you tips on other lifestyle changes that you can work into your daily or weekly routine.

Staying Motivated

Staying motivated while on a healthy eating lifestyle can be challenging sometimes, especially when you hit a weight-loss plateau (in which you are no longer able to lose weight) or when the holidays come around. Having an accountability partner and focusing on all the benefits that you are already seeing from your healthy eating lifestyle can help you stay on track. But what about in the beginning, when your whole body is sore from the toxins being purged from it and you don't think you will survive another sugar craving?

One necessary component of staying motivated is to make one change at a time rather than jumping in headfirst. Each time you make a change, be sure to replace the original with something even better. That way, you are easing yourself into a positive transition in which you actually like the replacement better; the changes will be much longer lasting than if you focus on deprivation and what you can't have. First, focus on eliminating sugar from your diet. Are you a heavy soda drinker? Start there. Throw out all the soda and get rid of all the excuses for needing it. No, you don't need to raise your blood sugar with a soda and no, you don't need the caffeine in it. Find a sugar-free alternative (not diet soda or anything that contains artificial sweeteners!). Kombucha is a fermented tea that still has a fizzy, slightly sweet taste but, unlike soda, has health-boosting probiotics, vitamins, and minerals. Many people have found that kombucha is a great alternative to soda. While it can be expensive to purchase (one bottle usually costs around three dollars), you can learn to make it at home for pennies a gallon.

Once the soda habit is gone, move on to your next sugar vice. Is it ice cream? A mid-afternoon crash that you solve with something sweet? Donuts? Find a suitable replacement for those things; instead of ice cream, use frozen bananas to make a smooth and creamy frozen snack. Eat frozen grapes; they can be a great way to satisfy a sweet tooth. For the mid-afternoon crash, plan ahead with a fruit salad that you will eat instead of going to the vending machine. Not only will you satisfy the need for something sweet, but you will have given your body an infusion of vitamins and minerals.

After a while, the gradual changes will start to snowball into a major lifestyle overhaul. Without you even thinking about it, that one vegan meal a day will become two. You'll want to take the stairs instead of the elevator because you love the feeling of getting the blood flowing. Give yourself enough choices, and you won't even miss the things that you thought you couldn't live without.

Habit Formation

Habits take between two weeks and one month to form. During the time when a habit is being formed, one slip-up can derail the entire process. The trick to forming a habit is to be aware of that fact so that you are equipped to not let those inevitable slip-ups get you completely off-track. Maybe you planned to go to the gym every Tuesday, Thursday, and Saturday. This Saturday, though, you just couldn't bring yourself to do it. Instead, you watched Netflix and ate grilled cheese sandwiches and drank soda. Before the end of the first season that you are binging on, you have convinced yourself that this healthy-eating lifestyle isn't for you and you can't do it, anyway. All of the efforts that you put into creating the necessary habits to enforce your lifestyle changes could easily be derailed at that point unless you are already aware of that potential.

The good news is that everybody has slip-ups. Everybody has bad days. And the best news is that that's perfectly OK! So, you had pizza delivered and ate four slices while going through two seasons of Game of Thrones instead of going to the gym. That does not make you a failure. It just means that you need to get up and start again tomorrow.

Be kind to yourself, let yourself have a bad day, and then get back on track.

One key to preventing those slip-ups from becoming a regular occurrence is to try to figure out what causes them. Are you an emotional eater? Maybe a particularly stressful event or just feeling overwhelmed, rather than your own lack of willpower, led to you downing a pint of ice cream. Keep a journal so that you can stay on track of what keeps you motivated (what enables you to stay strong on good days) and what leads to you having a splurge.

Thirty days of healthy eating and regular exercise is usually enough to enforce the new lifestyle. However, remember that the most long-lasting changes are those that come gradually, so if you aren't able to become an immediate vegan and stay on track for 30 days, it's probably because you're trying to do too much at once. Get off of sugar for 30 days, and you will find that you no longer even want sweets. Then get off all processed food for 30 days, and you will find that you only want food that is fresh and nutritious. Next, exercise regularly for 30 days. You will find that you want to do it every day! Congratulations. You just developed the necessary habits to stay on track.

Foods to Focus on

One key to staying on track is to keep your eyes on the foods that you can focus on; there are far more foods that you can eat to support a healthy diet and lifestyle than foods that can derail it. Focus on continually expanding your palate to include more of the great variety of natural, plant-based foods that can help lead to overall health and well-being. Focus on eating plant-based foods that are grown without agrichemicals, to ensure that those toxins don't end up inside your body.

Fiber is a nutrient that passes through the digestive system unaltered; however, it slows the absorption of sugar and keeps you feeling full longer. Foods that are high in fiber should be consumed consistently. This does not include processed foods that have fiber artificially added to them, like Metamucil crackers or fiber powder.

Rather, it refers to foods that are naturally high in fiber. Vegetables that are particularly high in fiber include celery, carrots, artichokes, Brussels sprouts, and broccoli. Fruits that are high in fiber include berries (raspberries, blackberries, strawberries, and blueberries), avocados, apples, oranges, and pears. The best part about eating fiber-rich fruit is that even though it is sweet enough to satisfy a sugar craving, the fiber in it keeps your blood sugar and insulin levels from spiking. To ensure that the fiber isn't destroyed, try to eat fruits and vegetables uncooked as much as possible.

Other foods that should be focused on are foods that are bright and colorful. While sweet potatoes are technically starches rather than vegetables, they have a nutrient profile that can rival most vegetables, while having a sweetness that can make them even more satisfying than white potatoes. Spirulina and chlorella are algae that are loaded with B vitamins; they make a great addition to smoothies. Turmeric is a bright yellow-orange seasoning that has health benefits so strong that it is superior to many medications! Experiment by using as many natural herbs and seasonings in your cooking as you can.

Work on continually expanding your palate to include more colorful fruits and vegetables. When you are first trying new ones, start by adding them to smoothies, soups, or salads so that you can adjust to the taste. You will find that there are plenty of foods that your taste buds are just waiting to discover and enjoy!

Foods to Avoid

On any healthy-eating plan, the first group of foods that should absolutely be avoided is anything that causes a spike in insulin levels. High insulin levels are behind many cases of obesity and disease, so keeping your insulin stable is necessary to getting your health back. Sugar, juice, white bread, soda, and pasta are just a few examples of insulin-spiking foods that should be avoided at all costs.

Lectins are substances found in plant proteins that can contribute to leaky gut syndrome, a condition in which the lining of the intestines becomes porous, allowing undigested food and toxins directly into the body. Virtually all foods contain lectins, so they cannot be completely avoided. However, some foods contain very high levels of lectins and should not be consumed. Beans and pulses, including kidney beans, navy beans, fava beans, lima beans, pinto beans, soybeans, mung beans, peas, and lentils are all high in lectins. Cooking destroys some of them, but not all. Grains and cereals, especially whole grains (because most of the lectins are found in the shell of the seed), are particularly high in lectins. These foods include barley, wheat, corn, rice, and wheat germ.

Genetically modified organisms (GMO food) should be avoided like the plague. Genetic modification alters the genome of an organism so that it is essentially a new breed that is not recognized in nature. The altered DNA can actually alter the DNA in your body's cells! In addition, GMOs are heavily sprayed with glyphosate, an herbicide that is known to cause cancer, hormonal disruptions, infertility, and a host of other health problems. In addition to the dangers GMOs pose to human health, they literally have the potential to completely destroy the planet. They inhibit biodiversity, which is crucial to healthy ecosystems. The glyphosate used to treat them has penetrated the water table, heavily contaminated the soil, and is wreaking havoc on marine and another animal life.

Supplements

Before considering taking supplements, remember that most of your nutritional needs should be met from the food that you eat. Supplements should be used only to enhance the nutritional benefits of food or to take the place of foods that you are unable to eat (for example, vegans often need to take supplements for the B complex). Use supplements in their most whole, natural form rather than chemically based supplements. For example, if you must use protein powder, use a brand that does not include chemicals in the powder and derives the protein from natural, rather than artificial, sources. Spirulina, chlorella, hemp, and chia seeds all make great supplements because they are entirely natural, come from plant-based sources, and can be added to food to make it more nutritious.

Some supplements can actually work adversely together to create a toxic brew in your blood. Talk to a doctor or pharmacist to ensure that any combination of supplements that you are taking is healthy.

CPSIA information can be obtained
at www.ICGtesting.com
Printed in the USA
LVHW030525061220
673433LV00015B/2480

9 789814 950060